The Sirtfood Diet

A Complete Beginner's Guide to Activate Your "Skinny Gene" for Easier and Longer-Lasting Weight Loss. Kick-Start Your Metabolism with Delicious Recipes and a 7-Day Meal Plan.

Kate Ross

Table of Contents

Introduction

The world has developed more in the last century than at any time previously in history. But, with this rapid development, people had to adapt to increased workloads and everyday stressors that most of our ancestors didn't know existed. With this increased workload and stress, people find it difficult to take the time to keep themselves healthy. There is a myriad of excuses that are made as to increasing waistlines and general lethargy. One of the most common of these excuses is people claiming that they don't have time to exercise and cook healthy meals, so they resort to whatever takeout option they're in the mood for.

In a person's adolescent years through to their early adult lives, they may find that they have a metabolism that allows them to eat whatever they desire and not put on any extra weight, but as one gets older, their metabolism starts to slow down, which comes with the terrible realization that you can't simply eat whatever you want to without worrying about the consequences. These poor diet choices will lead to problematic health complications later on in life, which can range from diabetes to hypertension—which will be detailed later in the book.

When people start to notice they are putting on the pounds, they tend to resort to fad diets to try and burn the excess fat that their body is storing, but many of these fad diets create more problems than many people tend to realize, and can be catastrophic to one's health.

The sirtfood diet, on the other hand, is not merely a fad diet and can be followed routinely without one developing unnecessary cravings. The sirtfood diet works so effectively because it focuses on increasing a person's plant-based food intake so the body can feel fuller while burning the necessary calories. Even though the sirtfood diet does focus on limiting calories, there are still additional food groups that can be consumed, like dark chocolate and red wine because they are so high in antioxidants.

One of the most effective ways for people to lose weight and keep it off is to ensure that their metabolism rates are boosted and remain increased permanently. This book will show you how to use the sirtfood diet effectively by incorporating a weekly eating plan that can be performed for 21 days with 24 easy and delicious sirtfood recipes. The sirtfood diet may restrict the number of calories that you consume on a daily basis, but you won't feel hungry when using this diet because of the amount of plant-based food items that you'll be consuming.

If you're worried that this is just another one of those diets that will leave you wanting more and just like all the others that have been attempted in the past, it may fall by the wayside very quickly... then you'll be pleasantly surprised when you realize how effective and how tasty the sirtfood meal-plan actually is. The famous singer/songwriter, Adele, lost more than 50 pounds while using the sirtfood diet and was very impressed with how effectively this diet-plan worked (Krstic, 2020). The world was in awe when Adele walked out on the set of Saturday Night Live (SNL), boasting her new and very attractive body. She was in better shape than ever and she wanted the world to see it.

The sirtfood meal-plan may feel like a diet at first, but as soon as one realizes how effective it is, it can quickly and easily become a lifestyle change. This is a tasty journey that everyone should try, even if you're at a healthy bodyweight because this meal-plan boosts metabolism and is filled with cancer-fighting antioxidants. This is definitely a meal-plan that won't disappoint.

Chapter 1: The Sirtfood Diet Explained

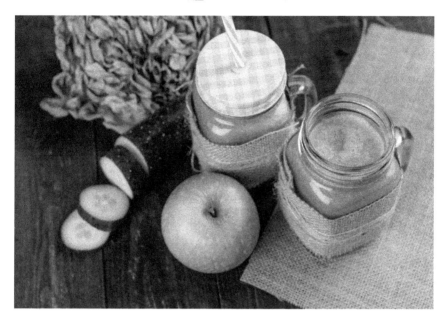

To fully understand how the sirtfood diet works, it first needs to be broken down into its fundamental elements. Most diets work in such a way that they restrict what foods a person can consume, and even though the sirtfood diet may be restrictive, it isn't as difficult to cope with as other restrictive diets and is definitely more effective.

The sirtfood diet was designed to activate a person's "skinny gene" and although that may sound a bit strange, it has everything to do with a person's metabolism. Once a person boosts their metabolism in a healthy way, then they'll naturally maintain healthy bodyweight for the rest of their lives. The two most effective ways of boosting your metabolism are through healthy eating and regular exercise. These two factors can work independently of one another, but they are much more effective when they're combined.

The sirtfood diet boosts a person's metabolism or activates their skinny gene by focusing on sirtuins. Sirtuins are a group of seven different proteins found in the human body, and these proteins have been found to regulate multiple bodily functions like inflammation, metabolism, and homeostasis.

The Science Behind Sirtuins

Sirtuins are groups of proteins that belong to the same family, and these proteins are responsible for regulating the health of cells and tissues within the body. These proteins help regulate the homeostasis within the body, which is the carefully regulated balance that keeps all of the organ systems in check and operating effectively.

Sirtuins may be a family of proteins, but they are different types of proteins that are more than just the proteins that are found in meat, beans, and protein shakes. These proteins work throughout the body's cells to ensure that all of the cells are functioning properly. The sirtuin proteins all have different functions, but they all work towards the ultimate balance of the body and effective functioning of all of the systems.

A person's body has approximately 60,000 different groups of proteins and sirtuins are only one of those familial groups. There are seven different sirtuins within body cells—three of the sirtuins are found within the mitochondria (the energy-giving parts of a cell), three of them work within the nucleus of the cell (where all of the genetic material is found), and one of them works in the cytoplasm of the cell, which, along with the cell membrane, maintains the structural integrity of the cell. The sirtuins are the proteins that help maintain the functionality of the cell by removing acetyl groups from other proteins.

Acetyl groups are in control of specific reactions within the body and the body's systems. Acetyl groups can be described as 'physical' tags on different protein groups. These physical tags allow for protein groups to react with each other. If proteins are like the departments within a cell, then the genetic material in the nucleus is like the CEO of the cell. The acetyl groups can then be described as the availability status of each department. This means that the acetyl group shows if specific proteins can work with sirtuins to cause specific reactions.

Sirtuins respond to and react with acetyl groups by going through a process known as deacetylation. This means that the sirtuins recognize the acetyl group on another protein molecule. The sirtuins then remove the acetyl group from that molecule, which then activates the molecule to perform the job that it needs to do.

The Discovery of Sirtuins

Sirtuins were first discovered in the mid-1970s by the geneticist, Amar Klar. He first identified sirtuins when he was observing the reproductive processes of yeast cells. He identified the specific sirtuin as the gene that allowed yeast cells to effectively reproduce with one another. Klar wasn't sure what to call these proteins, but he did continue to personally study them. After Klar made this discovery, research into sirtuins stagnated until the early 1990s began to develop once again. Researchers found that other protein genes were similar in structure, and they classified these homologous genes as sirtuins (Elysium Health n.d.).

One of the most interesting factors regarding sirtuins is that they are found across both plant and animal species. This was important to the research into sirtuins because of the potential functions that these protein genes were capable of. Sirtuin research has been largely connected to the aging process and metabolic activity, and since the 1990s, over 12,000 research papers have been released on sirtuins and their interactions.

What the Sirtfood Diet Is

Even though sirtuins aren't exactly the same as the proteins that are found in the foods that we eat, consuming certain products can allow for the body to produce more of these protein molecules naturally. Foods that are known to boost sirtuin levels in the body are known as 'sirtfoods.' Most of the foods that boost sirtuin levels in the body are plant-based and if you're a regular meat-eater, it may take some effort to follow this diet-plan strictly. That said, the overall effects of the sirtfood diet are definitely worth it.

The 20 foods that are the best sirtfoods will be included in the list below, and most of these ingredients will be included in the recipes in chapter 6:

- Red wine
- Kale and other leafy greens like spinach
- Onions
- Strawberries
- Fresh parsley
- Soy products
- Extra virgin olive oil (cold-pressed)
- Dark chocolate (85% cocoa and above)
- Buckwheat products
- Turmeric
- Matcha green tea
- Rocket

- Walnuts

- Chili products, particularly bird's eye chili

- Lovage leaves

- Fresh dates

- Blueberries

- Capers

- Coffee

- Red chicory

Combining these foods with a caloric intake that's relatively restrictive, the body naturally starts to produce more sirtuins. This diet's developers claim that the sirtfood diet will lead to rapid weight loss and healthy detoxification of the body, while maintaining healthy muscle tone and mass. This means that this diet can aid in combating the onset of chronic diseases and make people live much fuller lives.

This diet is very effective to help people lose weight but because it may be difficult to maintain this type of diet for long periods of time, there are ways that people can still increase their sirtuin count and metabolism even after the diet ends. There are certain boosters that will be discussed in the chapters to come that will help anyone maintain their weight loss regime.

The Effectiveness of The Sirtfood Diet

There has been much debate surrounding the "skinny gene" because it sounds like another fad diet solution. But, understanding how your metabolism works is one of the best ways for a person to maintain a healthy Body Mass Index (BMI) throughout their lives. The sirtfood diet boosts the metabolism and makes the body's cells healthier which enables them to combat metabolic and other chronic diseases from developing.

That said, there is some controversy surrounding the sirtfood diet because it's not as well researched as other diets, so the full extent of the effects isn't entirely known. But, there is sufficient evidence to prove that this diet does enable effective and healthy weight loss. Additionally, many of the foods that are on the list, although normally considered healthy, aren't fully researched to understand their health benefits. Hence, there haven't been any research studies performed on humans whether or not diets that promote sirtuin production are entirely beneficial.

Although there haven't been official research studies performed on the sirtfood diet, there have been several participants that have logged their weight-loss journey. Several participants that combined daily exercise with calorie-controlled sirtfood diets lost an average of seven pounds in their first week (Jones, 2020). But, these dieters only experienced this type of weight loss when they restricted their caloric intake to 1000 calories, which is considered a very low-calorie diet, but it's still enough to keep the metabolism from moving into a mode of starvation.

It's important to note that this diet can have negative effects on a person's weight loss. The reason for this is because people that choose to restrict the number of calories that they have on a daily basis will inadvertently lose weight, but their rapid weight loss can't be maintained like it is in the first couple of weeks and then they lose hope and revert back to their old ways. Additionally, when a person stays on a calorie-restricted diet, their body starts to burn excess fat and glycogen (stored glucose) to make up for the calories that they aren't receiving. This makes them lose large amounts of weight at the beginning of their diet process, but once their stores become depleted, their weight loss process starts to slow down.

When your body stores glucose in the form of glycogen, your body needs to store three to four water molecules for every glycogen molecule. This means that when glycogen is being burnt for energy, the body is also getting rid of "water weight" which makes the first few weeks in this process very impressive. In the first week of any diet that requires you to restrict your caloric intake, one-third of the weight that you lose comes from your stored glycogen and fat stores, while two-thirds comes directly from the stored water and some muscle mass in the body.

But, as soon as your caloric intake returns to normal, then the weight is put back on again because the body is trying to restore the glycogen stores that were completely depleted. The combination of putting weight back on when the diet ends, or slowing your metabolism because of the low intake of calories on a daily basis, can make one doubtful enough to rather avoid this type of diet.

That said, when used prudently, this type of diet can be very beneficial to one's health, overall well-being, and metabolism. But instead of sticking to an insanely low number of calories every day, it's better to consume slightly more calories on a daily basis using the sirtfood recipes that you're going to learn later. Doing this will make your weight-loss slower than it would be if you were only consuming 1000 calories per day, but because your body doesn't feel starved, then your metabolism will increase instead of decrease. Additionally, your body will be producing higher amounts of sirtuins which will maintain the health of all of your cells in your body.

Using the sirtfood diet while consuming a healthy number of calories every day is definitely the most effective and permanent solution to losing weight.

Chapter 2: The Benefits of the Sirtfood Diet

Because of the huge influx of fad diets, all of which promise world-changing effects, it's difficult to know which diets can actually be effective. One of the most difficult aspects of any diet is being hit with a craving when you least expect it. Cravings occur in restrictive diets because the body feels like it's starving and it will start craving foods that are higher in calories to help replenish the stores that are being depleted quickly. To understand why some diets work while others don't, it's important to understand how the body works and a person can still gain weight even when they feel they don't eat enough.

The body's metabolism is the energy-producing factory in the body. When the body is regularly fueled and exercised, then the metabolism knows that it can safely be at an increased rate because the body is replenished soon after energy stores are used. This means that the metabolism doesn't need many energy stores in the factory. The primary problem with heavily restricting the number of calories that you consume in a day is that your body feels stressed that it isn't going to receive enough fuel, so it stores as much as it can whenever it's fed.

The reason for this is twofold. First, the metabolism itself slows down to store as much energy as it possibly can in the form of glycogen and body fat. And, second, when a person is stressed, whether it's physiologically or emotionally, their bodies will release hormones with this stress response.

The two main hormones that are associated with a stress response are adrenaline and cortisol. Adrenaline is released in times of immediate stress like dangerous situations. Adrenaline produces a fight, flight, or freeze response. When adrenaline is released into the bloodstream from the adrenal glands, the response is practically immediate—the heart rate spikes to pump oxygen to the major organs and muscles for quick movement. The lungs expand rapidly to bring in as much air as possible in case one needs to run away quickly, the pupils expand to let in as much light as possible towards the retina so that one can see in dark places, and sometimes incontinence can occur because a body can move much faster without urine or feces weighing them down.

The second hormone, cortisol, also works in stressful situations, but these are more prolonged stressful situations like when the body is starving. In situations where the body starts to starve the body releases cortisol because it can feel the physical stress of starvation. This physical stress causes the body to seek any way possible to preserve all of the energy that it can by slowing its metabolic rate. Cortisol is the hormone that does exactly that—it slows the metabolism and allows for the body to store as much energy as it can in the forms of glycogen and body fat.

Unfortunately, our bodies aren't able to differentiate what type of stress we are feeling. With the hectic lifestyles and career choices that many people have in today's day and age, the release of cortisol is frequently seen in people with high-stress jobs. Many people that have these types of careers find it incredibly difficult to lose weight, even though they try as many diets as they can. Their bodies just seem to be against them… if you find yourself in this category, then don't fret, because there is a solution.

The stress of everyday life won't go anywhere, but there are ways that you can use to decrease the effects of the stress and keep your metabolism where it's supposed to be. Cortisol will lower your metabolism, so it's important to use regular eating and exercise habits to keep your metabolism and BMI in check. Most of the people that recommend sirtfood diet variations, recommend that you consume no more than 1000 calories per day, but this isn't a long-term solution. The foods that promote sirtuin production in the body are generally healthy and healthy amounts of these calories can be consumed every day to make this more of a long-term lifestyle choice, than a short-term "crash diet."

Appetite Control

One of the greatest problems that people find when they're trying to lose weight is that they are constantly hungry. This hunger may not necessarily be the fact that they're hungry, but it may be the reason because they're restricting their bodies and this makes them constantly peckish. The problem with this is that even though people have the capacity to portray the type of will-power needed to make these types of restrictive diets work, it can't be a long-term solution without learning how to control your appetite.

It may be tempting to buy appetite suppressants from your local drug-store, but the long-term effects of those types of medications can be very detrimental, so it's better to do it the natural way. The first way to control your appetite is by consuming sirt foods that are higher in plant-based fiber and proteins. Consuming these products will help make you feel fuller for longer, even though you're getting the same number of calories compared to having the same product in a juiced form.

The second way to control your appetite is by eating small snacks regularly, this does go against the normal teachings of the sirtfood diet, but this is the best way to maintain your metabolism and keep it burning the energy that you're putting into your body instead of storing it. Eating smaller portions regularly is the best way to control your appetite and to control any unexpected cravings.

The third way to control your appetite is by drinking enough liquids throughout the day. This may be a temporary fix, but those that drink enough water and green juice (this will be discussed later) will control random urges to suddenly stuff food into their mouths.

It may be tempting to find other ways to suppress your appetite, especially if you know that you struggle with impulse control, but there are much healthier and effective ways to keep your hunger at bay. Fortunately, using the sirtfood diet effectively will help you maintain your hunger pangs and it will become easier with time. Remember, if you're giving your body everything and all the nutrients that it needs, then it won't have any reason to crave things that are outside of the food that it's getting.

Activating Your Skinny Gene

Truthfully, no one was meant to be obese, or even overweight for that matter. So, finding the right type of meal plan is needed to maintain a healthy body. Unfortunately, many fad diets that people think are quick fixes may be detrimental to their bodies even though they make them lose weight.

The best way for a person to lose weight and keep it off is by activating their skinny gene. This doesn't actually have anything to do with genetics but has a lot more to do with making one's body believe that it's receiving enough energy throughout the day that it doesn't need to store any of it because it's receiving enough from the ingested foods.

The overall effect of boosting your metabolism in a healthy way is that it stays boosted even after you stop your diet. The problem with practically all fad diets is that they seem to fail as soon as a person stops their diet and returns back to normal eating. This, inadvertently, makes them gain the weight back that they lost. When using the sirtfood diet without restricting your daily caloric intake to less than 1000, and instead of keeping it to between 2300 and 2500 calories per day, then your metabolism will stay boosted after other foods are reintroduced into the mix after the first few weeks of the strict sirtfood diet.

Fighting Chronic Diseases and Their Onsets

One of the greatest causes of chronic diseases in today's world is the sheer amount of unhealthy foods that people consume far too regularly. People find many excuses to eat junk food, and although many of them may be legitimate, they are still detrimental to one's health. Fast-foods are filled with hidden saturated and trans-fatty acids, salt, and refined sugars and these products do increase the risk of developing chronic diseases.

Three of the most prolific chronic diseases that are known today that can be linked to unhealthy diets are hypercholesterolemia (high cholesterol), hypertension (high blood pressure), and diabetes. The high cholesterol levels are caused by the number of unhealthy fatty-acids that are hidden in junk-foods, hypertension is directly linked to the amount of salt that people consume on a daily basis, and diabetes is linked to the amount of sugar that is unnecessarily added to many food products. There are genetic factors that can play a role in these chronic diseases, but they are hugely affected by the amount of unhealthy eating that far too many are drawn to.

Research has found that replacing diets that are low in fiber and high in saturated fats with diets that promote sirtuin production in the body, will allow for a greatly decreased risk of developing these chronic diseases (Pallauf, 2013). The reason for this is three-fold:

First, the sirtuin production from the sirtfood diet will strengthen the cells in the body and make them less susceptible to damage from oxidative stress. The increased rate of repair in practically all of the body cells will help reduce the risk of developing any of these chronic diseases in the future.

Second, since many of these foods are higher in insoluble fiber than other processed foods, they lower the amount of cholesterol that's absorbed into the bloodstream by binding it in the intestines and passing it out in the feces.

Third, these types of foods allow the metabolism to accelerate naturally because they're promoting healthy cellular function. As soon as a person consumes foods that produce sirtuin production in the body, the metabolism naturally increases. This is one of the primary reasons why eating enough calories in the sirtfood diet is important because it will boost your metabolism and keep it accelerated.

Sleeping Better

Many people might be overweight because of unhealthy eating habits, but one of the most detrimental factors that can affect a person is unhealthy sleeping habits. Research has found that one in three people suffer from insomnia and many of these cases are worsened by unhealthy diets (Sleep Health Foundation, n.d.).

It's imperative to understand that what we put into our bodies will determine how we function. People that lead unhealthy lifestyles won't sleep as well as those that regularly exercise and eat healthy meals. This may not seem overly important but sleep is one of the most vital factors of maintaining one's metabolism. The reason for this is because people that don't sleep well put extra physiological stress on their bodies, which puts them at higher risk of developing chronic diseases like the ones mentioned in the section prior.

It's important for an adult to regularly maintain a sleeping pattern of between six and eight hours of sleep a night. Anything less than this will eventually lead to problematic physiological outcomes. The sirtfood diet helps people sleep better because it requires people's bodies to work harder to digest their meals and get a lower calorie-count afterward. This may seem counterintuitive, but having one's body work harder for the nutrients in the food that's given to it isn't a bad thing.

The sirtfood diet is filled with foods that are rich in insoluble fiber, and because these are difficult to digest, they may burn more calories than they offer when digested—this works wonders in any weight-loss program. Additionally, because your body is working harder to digest the food that it's consuming, it will feel more tired at the end of the day. This enables people to sleep better and is one of the major benefits of the sirtfood diet.

If you have trouble sleeping, as many people do, it is necessary to promote healthy sleeping habits during your sirtfood diet routine. Using the sirtfood diet will help you sleep better, especially if you're exercising, but there are other ways to maximize your sleep. The reason why it's important to not neglect your sleep is that healthy sleeping patterns are imperative for the body to heal and maintain its metabolism.

First, it's imperative that you make your sleeping environment as conducive to sleep as possible. Any distractions should be removed from the bedroom, which includes technological distractions. The bedroom should be reserved for three things only, namely sleep, reading, and sex. All other activities should be done elsewhere because your mind will automatically start to move to those distractions when you're trying to get a good night's rest.

Second, it's important to calm your mind before bed. Any stressors from the day need to be, ideally, left outside of the bedroom for you to focus on falling asleep. Of course, concentrating on falling asleep can be counterintuitive because it may very well be the thing that keeps you from falling asleep. But, having mental techniques to fall asleep quickly is the best way to maintain a healthy body and mind. These techniques include meditation, and focusing on thinking as little as possible until sleep comes. When you think about as little as possible, you will fall asleep much faster than you usually would.

Third, it's important not to eat any food an hour before bed. In the sirtfood meal-plans, dinners are normally smaller than other meals, but nevertheless, it's important not to have your digestive system working while you're trying to fall asleep. People that eat right before bed tend to wake up feeling rather groggy and lethargic, and the reason for this is because the body has been working while it was meant to be resting. This creates a repetitive cycle of exhaustion and does wreak havoc on the metabolism.

The sirtfood diet will help you sleep better because your body is going to be repairing a lot of the damage that was previously inflicted. This cellular repair is going to need sleep for additional aid, and this will make you more sleepy at night. This is the primary reason why the sirtfood diet helps in creating healthy sleep cycles. If, however, you still don't sleep well, then it's important to use other mental techniques to relax before bed because that will also help your metabolism.

Chapter 3: The Sirtfood Diet Ingredients

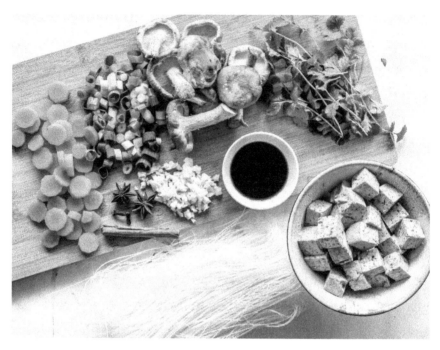

This chapter is going to discuss the different food groups that you should consume in this diet and why they're important. It's needed to find a balance, and although there may be some ingredients on this list that you may not be partial towards, you do need to keep as much variety as possible in any meal-plan that you want to use. People that become bored with their meal-plans will revert back to unhealthy eating habits. Variety is key to success for the mind and the body.

Red Wine

This may seem like the most attractive part of this diet because most diets strictly forbid alcohol, and one's that allow them, instantly seem more appealing to many people. Red wine is definitely one of the alcohols that should be considered for semi-regular consumption. The reason for this is because red wine is filled with antioxidants, and it not only lowers blood pressure, but research has shown that it can be beneficial in naturally lowering blood sugar levels (Davis, 2017). This satisfying, velvety, red drink is on this list because it's one of the alcoholic beverages that promote sirtuin production in the body.

That said, it's important to note, that although red wine is packed with health benefits, it does need to be taken in moderation and on semi-regular occasions. The reason for this is because red wine is still alcoholic, and alcohol can affect people's sleep negatively and it does have a fair number of calories—approximately 85 calories per 250ml glass. It's important for everyone wanting to go on this diet to use any alcoholic beverages responsibly. Healthy intake is around one glass for women and two glasses for men in a single sitting. The reason why there's a difference between men and women is two-fold.

First, men generally weigh more than women and have a larger muscle mass. This increased muscle mass contains a lot of water, which helps counteract the effects of alcohol. Second, men have a hormone in their stomach-linings known as alcohol dehydrogenase, which is a hormone that aids in breaking down alcohol before it enters the bloodstream. These two factors do allow men to drink slightly more than their female counterparts, but it's still healthier for them to have on the lower end of the scale.

Kale, Spinach, and Rocket

It's well-known that green, leafy vegetables are high in vitamin K and iron, but there's a lot more to these food items than just those two variables. These vegetables are packed full of fiber and antioxidants, making them some of the best preventers of not only colon cancers but general cancerous cells as well.

Including these vegetables into your sirtfood diet is a must because they also help stimulate sirtuin production in the cells, and combined with the number of antioxidants that they have within them, they truly are some of the best inclusions in the sirtfood diet, or any diet for that matter.

These vegetables are low in calories and require a lot of effort to digest, so it's important not to eat them within an hour of going to bed, but these make delicious lunch-time options, and they're very easy to whip up when there isn't much time left in the mornings. Some people have favorites among these leafy vegetables, and even though you will probably gravitate towards one of them, it's important to have a variety of these vegetables to keep from getting bored and gaining all of the benefits of different green vegetables.

Onions / Red Onions

Onions are not only great additions to food and enhance the flavor of the meal, but they also have several health-boosting benefits. Onions are known to boost immunity and this allows people to stay healthier in times when viral infections are spreading between people. These root vegetables are high in antioxidants and have many antibacterial properties. Because of their capabilities to heal, they are also known to enhance sirtuin production, so including them into your diet is a great way to boost your health and your metabolism.

Onions can be consumed raw or cooked according to your own personal preference. Obviously, most people prefer to have it cooked and even though some of the nutrients and antioxidants are destroyed during the cooking process, they are still remarkably beneficial to eat when cooked.

Berries

Practically all berries are very high in vitamin C, which is one of the most powerful antioxidants known to man, and other vitamins and minerals. These little superfoods are a great addition to anyone's diet plan. The most effective of the berries in the sirtfood diet are strawberries and blueberries, because of the sheer percentage of antioxidants that they have in them.

Berries are great to snack on because of their size, but they're also great to make smoothies out of. It is important to remember that smoothies can be high in calories, so it's important to carefully choose the ingredients before making it, because a smoothie can easily make you exceed your daily calorie-limit if you aren't careful.

Dark Chocolate

Another great addition to the sirtfood diet is definitely dark chocolate, but the type of dark chocolate is vitally important here. Sweet chocolates aren't going to have the health benefits of chocolates with high cocoa content. The reason for this is because cocoa is divided into cocoa powder and cocoa butter. Milk and white chocolates use cocoa butter for the majority of their productions, and although this gives the chocolate a rich and creamy texture, it's not nearly as healthy as the chocolates that are higher in the powdered aspect of the cocoa bean.

Practically all of the fat from the cocoa bean is found in the cocoa butter and although many people don't like the bitterness of cocoa powder, it's packed with antioxidants and metabolism-boosting properties. Chocolates that are under 85% cocoa shouldn't be consumed because they won't be beneficial to the weight loss process or the production of sirtuins within the cells. Additionally, chocolates that are higher in cocoa will have less sugar than lower percentages and this will lower the overall calorie count of the chocolate. It's worth it to go for chocolates with the highest cocoa percentage.

Besides, having a glass of red wine while intermittently having a bite of dark chocolate is very satisfying. These two items complement each other and can be used as a 'dessert' on days when you have a few calories to spare.

Turmeric and Chili Products

Research has found that people that eat spicy foods temporarily boost their metabolisms by around 8% (O'Conner, 2006). Even though this boost isn't permanent, it's still worthwhile to boost your metabolism in short bursts. Additionally, spices like turmeric and chili products are high in vitamin C and other antioxidants, making them vital to combat oxygen-free radicals and other cancer-causing molecules in the body.

These products can be taken in several different ways. Some people do struggle with spicy foods, but there are ways that these substances can still be taken without burning your mouth. Many homeopathic stores sell these spices as supplements in capsule or tablet forms, so that they can be taken without the discomfort in one's mouth.

If you, on the other hand, enjoy spicy foods, then it's a great idea to utilize these spices on a regular basis because they don't have much in the way of calories, and do have a lot of antioxidants. They also add great flavor to food, so it's prudent to start introducing these spices little-by-little until you're used to a little more heat in your food.

Matcha Green Tea and Coffee

Matcha tea is definitely the new kid on the block when it comes to health drinks, but its popularity has skyrocketed in recent years. Just like the original green tea, matcha tea comes from the same plant, but it's grown slightly differently and has a rather different profile to the original green tea.

When farmers grow matcha, they cover the plants for 30 days before they harvest them. This drastically increases the chlorophyll production in the plants, which gives it a much darker tone. This increased level of chlorophyll works as a powerful antioxidant in the body. Once the plants are harvested, the leaves are carefully removed from their stems before being ground into a fine green powder known as matcha. This fine powder contains all of the beneficial nutrients of the tea leaf, which results in much higher forms of caffeine and antioxidants when compared to normal green tea.

Studies have shown that the antioxidants found in matcha can help protect the liver, aid in weight loss, and protect the heart from previous damage caused by unhealthy lifestyle habits (Link, 2020). There are other benefits to consuming matcha on a semi-regular basis, and one of them is an increased level of brain function because of the amount of unrefined caffeine that's available in the powdered leaves.

Coffee, on the other hand, may seem like a strange addition to this list—even more so than wine or chocolate, because many people believe that coffee isn't as healthy as other drinks, but this isn't exactly true. Coffee in its purest form is filled with caffeine and antioxidants (much like matcha tea), and it can be used for the benefit of anyone that chooses this supplement when used correctly.

Caffeine may be a stimulant, but it also boosts the metabolism when taken in the correct dosages. Excessive intakes of caffeine are detrimental to a person's well-being, but in moderate doses, the effects can truly benefit a person. The antioxidants found in coffee beans stimulate sirtuin production within the cell, which helps in lowering the risk of developing cancerous cells from developing.

Coffee can be addictive and many people do consume too much of this product, however, when taken prudently, there are many health benefits associated with it. Both matcha tea and coffee are worthwhile supplements in the sirtfood diet and should be taken every couple of days.

Chapter 4: The Sirtfood Diet Plan

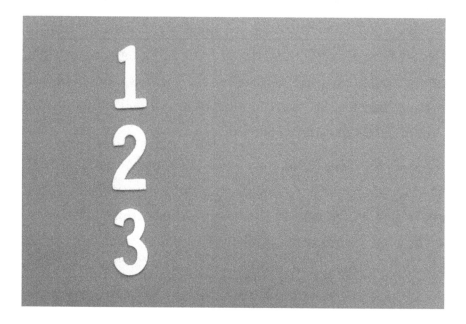

There are many fad diets that promise results if you follow certain regimes, but the sirtfood diet is divided into three phases where you can judge whether or not the diet is working for you. The first two phases are the primary phases and they will last you a minimum of 21 days. You may feel that this needs to be adjusted, but 21 days is the best amount of time for you to introduce the sirtfood diet into your lifestyle routine.

Once the 21 days are over, then you can move into a more permanent form of 'sirtifying' your meals, where you add extra food groups into your daily meals to ensure that you ingest adequate amounts of sirtuin-boosting foods. For the primary two phases, you will need to go to the nearest grocery store and pick up a few items that were mentioned previously. But, it's important to note that some of these items can be rather expensive, especially when one wants to purchase items like matcha tea because it can be costly in some stores.

Another cost that you're going to need to consider purchasing is a juicer, and if you think that your smoothie-maker will do the trick then you're mistaken... you need a juicer. The reason for this is because you are going to need to make the "Sirtfood Diet Green Juice", which is packed full of the nutrients that you need and it will be one of the tastiest additions to this diet.

This green juice is going to become one of the most important factors of this whole diet because it's going to kickstart your metabolism and make you lose weight quickly in the first few weeks. This occurs because it helps the body burn glycogen, but also some of the ingredients in this juice are natural diuretics and it will promote the excretion of excess water retention.

The Green Sirtfood Juice

Since this juice is going to become a regular part of your daily routine, it will be wise to stock up on all of the items that you need to make this juice in advance. Because it works out much more cost-effective this way. The ingredients that you will need are:

1. 2½ to 3 ounces (75 to 90 grams) of fresh kale leaves. You can leave the stalks attached to the leaves because you're juicing them, but do ensure that they're adequately cleaned before putting them through the juicer.

2. 1 to 2 ounces (30 to 60 grams) of fresh rocket.

3. Roughly 5 grams (0.20 ounces of a small handful) of fresh parsley, because it adds to the fresh flavor of the juice and it's packed with antioxidants. Only forgo the parsley if absolutely needed.

4. 2 to 3 large celery sticks. Celery is a great addition to any weight loss program because celery is considered a negative-calorie food item. This means that celery requires more energy to digest than it gives to the body, so it accelerates the weight-loss goal.

5. 5 to 10 grams (0.20 to 0.35 ounces) of fresh ginger. Ginger is one of those spices that needs to be consumed regularly because it's packed with so much goodness. The antioxidants and healing qualities of ginger make it one of the most valuable spices in a person's kitchen.

6. 1 large green apple.

7. 1 whole lemon (half will suffice if it's too sour for your liking).

8. ½ a teaspoon of matcha green tea powder.

Juice all of these ingredients together, barring the matcha tea powder because you can just mix that into the juice at the end, and drink while fresh. This juice can be made ahead of time, but it's imperative that you seal the container/bottle sufficiently to prevent any of the fridge air from getting into the container and affecting the juice.

The First Phase

The beginning stage of any diet is one of the most vital aspects because this is the period that people are going to lose the most weight because of the burning of glycogen and the loss of water weight. The first phase in the sirtfood diet lasts an entire week, and it does involve calorie restriction (this is where the green juice comes into play). The original sirtfood diet was intended to help people lose around seven pounds in their first week of the diet, but this isn't a healthy form of weight loss because the weight is inevitably put back on again after the diet ends.

It's better to restrict yourself to around 2500 calories per day (instead of 1000 calories) and lose weight more gradually. Using this type of method will enable your body to readjust its metabolism instead of shocking it, and this will result in a more permanent weight loss program. For the first three days in the sirtfood diet, it recommended that people only eat one meal a day and drink three glasses of green juice. This diet is attractive to people because they can choose any meal from sirtfood recipes as long as they don't exceed 1000 calories.

Days four through seven increase the number of calories to 1500 with two green juices every day. This adjustment allows for a remarkable weight loss program. However, this type of shock treatment is difficult for the body to adapt to, and even though it's tempting to want to drop so many pounds in the first week of a diet, it's not a sustainable form of weight loss. Remember that more gradual weight loss using the sirtfood diet-plan is much more effective in the long run.

The Second Phase

The second phase lasts for a minimum of two weeks but can be extended to three if you're feeling like your body is handling the effects of the diet. The second phase doesn't have an absolute calorie limit and meals can be increased to three times a day while consuming at least one green juice every day. This meal-plan can be personalized, which makes it attractive to many people. Controlling your intake of calories is important, but healthy weight loss is even more so, so do so gradually!

There are a variety of meals that can be included in this phase and many of them will be discussed in the chapters to come, but it's important to adjust your meal-plan accordingly and balance it carefully. Keep in mind that if you get bored with foods, your body will feel the same way, so if you dedicate your time and energy to eat three kale salads a day for three whole weeks, you will inevitably fail... probably after the first few days, because people can only eat so much kale before they become completely bored with it. Variety is definitely key here, just like it is in the lives that we lead. Monotony becomes boring and it will lead to a person giving up on what they're doing, no matter how good their intentions were at the beginning of their journeys.

If you're aiming to look after your body and get healthy during this process, then you're going to want to enjoy it as much as possible. Those that choose to see their diet journeys as punishments or just to get the bodies that they want won't go as far as they'd like, and most of the time, will fail. This process is meant to be enjoyed.

The Third Phase

The first two phases can be repeated as regularly as you desire, and changing things from time to time will help your body lose more weight because your metabolism is required to adapt according to the diet plan that you're on. The third phase of this diet plan has everything to do with returning to normal after the diet is finished.

It's vitally important to remember that most diets don't work because people see diets as diets. Diets have expiration dates and once they've reached their goals, they feel that they can just return to normal and carry on with their old eating habits. This is one of the worst decisions that anyone can make after a diet because diets do deplete glycogen stores and then returning the higher calorie diets will allow for the body to replenish the glycogen that is lost. If the body feels like it's starving then it will take all of the extra calories that are given to it and store it away for later. This is why a gradual form of weight loss will offer the most permanent solution.

In this third phase of your sirtfood diet, it's recommended that you start 'sirtifying' your meals by adding in sirtfoods on a very regular basis. It's not possible for someone to be on a diet forever, but it is possible to have a lifestyle change. Choosing to eat healthier and focussing on consuming foods that are higher in antioxidants and promote sirtuin production is the healthiest way to go.

Common Mistakes

As with any big decisions in life, it's necessary to do the planning beforehand. Those that choose to go on a journey like this half-heartedly will inevitably fail because it's tougher than people realize. Even though it's recommended that you don't go as extreme as limiting yourself to only 1000 or 1500 calories a day, 2500 calories are still much lower than many people consume.

This will become difficult, and if you become hungry, it's very easy to decide to rather give up and not carry on with the diet plan.

It will take the necessary mental strength to accomplish this journey, and even though many people have been successful while using the sirtfood diet, it still took a lot of determination for them to succeed.

If you want to succeed in using this diet for yourself, then you will need to make the decision for yourself and you need to remind yourself why you're doing it. People that are forced into diets don't make it because they didn't make the decision for themselves. But, those that chose to lose weight and become healthier often find themselves succeeding. A diet may be a physical game, but it's also very much a mental game. A person who's mentally strong will stick to what they decide and will make a difference for themselves.

If, however, you're not mentally strong and you know that you struggle with self-control, then it's important to develop a buddy-system where you're accountable to someone else. Having someone to lean on when you're struggling does make the world of difference.

Finally, when starting this diet, don't necessarily see it as a diet, because diets are unappealing and just the sound of them can make a person feel depressed. But, once a person decides to make a lifestyle change, then they stick to their goals, because even if they fall off the wagon and eat meals that are made out of junk-food, they don't feel completely deflated and that all of their hard work has been undone. Lifestyles changes are easier to stick to than diet-plans.

Frequently Asked Questions About the Sirtfood Diet

This section is included because many people have doubts about things that they're not entirely sure of, and if you're a person that likes to be fully prepared and informed before making a decision, then these are the most frequently asked questions about the sirtfood diet.

Have Sirtfoods Become the New Superfoods?

There's no question about whether or not sirtfoods are good for you because they're mostly highly nutritious, filled with antioxidants, and very high in plant-based fiber. Research has found that these foods have been linked to a myriad of different types of health benefits (Jones, 2020). For example, very dark chocolate is filled with antioxidants that reduce inflammation in the body and lower the chances of developing heart disease. Green tea and matcha tea lowers blood pressure and reduces the risk of developing type II diabetes and having strokes and other cerebral events.

Practically all of the sirtfoods that are described in this book have remarkable health benefits in people. However, the research into boosting sirtuins in the body through eating the right types of foods is still in its preliminary stages. But, there have been tests performed in animal subjects that were presented with sirtfoods, and their cellular strengthening was very noticeable (Jones, 2020). The same researchers also noticed that worms, yeast, and mice that were exposed to sirtfoods lived longer than their normal counterparts.

Additionally, when a person has been on the sirtfood diet and they're producing higher levels of sirtuins, their bodies burn more fat in times of calorie-restriction or fasting. They're also more sensitive to the insulin that's released from their pancreas. A research study in mice has proven that higher levels of sirtuins do result in fat being burned faster than average (Jones, 2020).

There have been additional theories that because sirtuins can aid in anti-inflammatory processes, they may be able to slow down and even prevent the development of Alzheimer's disease and other cognitive problems. But, these haven't been proven yet and research is still being conducted around this.

Sirtuins may prolong life in mice and other animals, but there haven't been any confirmations of this fact in human trials. It's still unknown if the increase in sirtuins can prevent cancer and other chronic illnesses from developing, but the understanding behind these theories is positively hopeful.

Is the Sirtfood Diet Sustainable and Healthy?

There are many fad diets that promise quick and effective weight loss, and even though this may be true, some of them can be very detrimental to one's overall health and well-being. The sirtfood diet is primarily made up of healthy foods, so it's simple to assume that there won't be any health complications with this diet, but some caution does need to be exhibited with this diet. The reason for this is because eating a few healthy food items on a daily basis might not meet the nutritional needs of your body, and it can result in malnutrition if extreme calorie-restriction is performed for too long periods of time.

The original sirtfood diet is dangerously restrictive, and most professionals don't advise that anyone restricts themselves to only 1000 calories per day without the close supervision of a trained professional or physician. Even 1500 calories can be considered far too low for most people, so it can be dangerous to try and sustain that number of calories for long periods of time.

One of the reasons why it's dangerous to restrict yourself to such a low number of calories is that it can affect your body's pH balance. Most people's bodies remain at a neutral pH balance of 7.40, but any fluctuations in this can be very detrimental to one's health. Restricting the number of calories that you put into your body affects the pH balance because the body is required to burn its fat stores for its primary energy. The fats, or ketones in a person's body lower the body's pH when burned for fuel and make the body more acidic. This can result in physical sickness and extreme discomfort.

Furthermore, the sirtfood diet requires people to drink three green juices per day in the first week of this diet and although that seems like a way to get in a lot of nutrients quickly, there are still hidden sugars in the juice. These sugars are found in the form of fructose and can be found in the apple and matcha powder. Although fructose is considered a fruit-sugar, it is still sugar. The reason why most people don't consume too many fructose in a single-sitting is that they consume the fiber of the fruit along with the fructose. This makes them fuller before they eat too much. Unfortunately, juice doesn't have the fiber content of the fruit or vegetables themselves and this can make a person consume too much fructose. This can spike a person's blood sugar levels and it can make them feel very unwell in the first week of the diet, especially if they're calorie-restricting.

Another concern about the sirtfood diet is that it's primarily plant-based, and although plant-based diets are easily sustainable, the foods that are considered sirtfoods are severely lacking in protein. This will affect the body severely if protein is withheld from it for long periods of time because the body will start to break down muscle fibers because it doesn't have the building blocks to repair any damage caused to them during everyday life.

Another factor that some people have a problem with is that it can become expensive to maintain. Buying a juicer and the ingredients to make juices regularly can become a costly affair after a few weeks. This is one of the reasons why people have fallen short of completing their diet plan, they just couldn't afford it anymore.

Overall, the idea behind this diet is great and it can be done healthily, but it does need to be seen more as a lifestyle change compared to a diet. This includes eating fewer calories a day but not having extreme restrictions on the number of calories that you do consume. This lifestyle change can be effective, but it needs to be done safely to lower the risk of developing health complications along the way. It would be terribly ironic if a person wants to lose weight and become healthy but they cause health problems to themselves because they implemented the diet-plan incorrectly.

This means that the original sirtfood diet isn't sustainable for long periods of time, in fact, even three weeks might be too long of a stretch. However, if this diet-plan is adapted and these foods are introduced on a daily basis, then it will be much more sustainable.

What Side Effects Can I Experience with the Sirtfood Diet?

Any type of diet is going to cause some side effects, especially in the beginning stages. When a person's body is used to receiving a specific number of calories every day, the first day of a new diet is going to come as a bit of a shock to the body, because psychologically and physically, people struggle with change. The first few days are also going to be a form of detox for the body and this is going to make you feel a little unwell. You might experience bouts of nausea and light-headedness, but these symptoms are fleeting and completely normal.

Even though this diet is more restrictive than others, it doesn't have the same side effects as other diet-plans, and as long there aren't underlying health issues like diabetes, then most of the side effects associated with the sirtfood diet are relatively easy to handle. It's important to note that if you do suffer from a chronic illness it's vital that you run through these diet-plans with your doctor first. Restrictive diets can be detrimental to someone with diabetes, and it can result in life-threatening complications if not used correctly.

Chapter 5: The Sirtfood Lifestyle Meal Plan

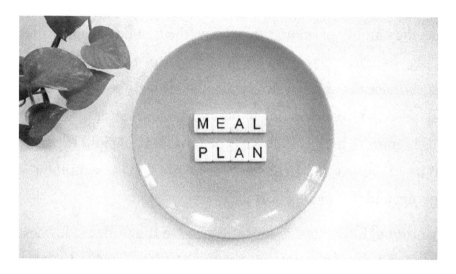

The meal plan that's going to be introduced here is going to be given over a three-week period and can be changed accordingly to what you feel you need to adjust. Since the sirtfood diet that you're going to follow is going to be more of a lifestyle change, then it's important to remember that everything that you do needs to be considered to be done for the long-term.

The recipes and meal plans in the next two chapters are going to include a balance of carbohydrates, proteins, healthy fats, and sirtuin-producing vegetables. Finding a healthy balance between all of the food groups will allow you to boost your metabolism and lose weight healthily. Do keep in mind that the crash sirtfood diet where you severely restrict yourself will make you lose weight very quickly, but that isn't a lifestyle that can be maintained. Slow and steady will win the race and you will manage to keep the weight off if you find a healthy balance in your eating habits.

It's also important to eat regularly. Starving yourself slows your metabolism and it will make your body feel stressed enough to start storing the energy as fat and glycogen. This is something that you want to avoid when you're trying to lose weight.

An example week is included in this chapter so that you can start to make your own meal plans. Only a one-week example is included because unlike the original sirtfood diet, this one has the same calorie count for all three weeks, which is 2500 calories per day—anything less than that is detrimental to the body and the metabolism.

The Meal Plan for Your Journey

The first week is going to be the hardest, because your body, most likely, isn't going to be used to the high levels of antioxidants being given to it. Even though I mentioned in the previous section that the green juices may have a fair amount of fructose in them, using them concurrently while eating smaller meals and snacks is a great way to balance out those sugars. All of the meals that are mentioned here will be detailed in the next chapter on their recipes and what you'll need to make them.

Monday

- Breakfast: Scrambled eggs and mushrooms
- Snack: Green juice
- Lunch: Kale salad with turmeric chicken and a honey and lime dressing
- Snack: Fresh strawberries, and celery sticks
- Dinner: King prawn stir fry with buckwheat noodles
- Dessert: A glass of red wine and a block of very dark, bitter chocolate

Tuesday

- Breakfast: The sirtfood style muesli
- Snack: Green juice
- Lunch: Baked salmon salad with mint dressing
- Snack: Green juice
- Dinner: A fragrant Asian hotpot
- Dessert: A glass of red wine and a block of very dark, bitter chocolate

Wednesday

- Breakfast: Smoked salmon and spinach omelet
- Snack: Celery and carrot sticks
- Lunch: Chicken, kale, and buckwheat noodles with a miso dressing
- Snack: Green juice

- Dinner: The simple chicken salad
- Dessert: A glass of red wine and a block of very dark, bitter chocolate

Thursday

- Breakfast: Chocolate chip granola cereal
- Snack: Green juice
- Lunch: Baked turmeric salmon
- Snack: Green juice
- Dinner: Buckwheat with kale and red onion dahl
- Dessert: Raspberry and blackcurrant jello

Friday

- Breakfast: The melon and grape sirt-juice
- Snack: Green juice
- Lunch: Avocado and buckwheat pasta salad
- Snack: Celery and carrot sticks
- Dinner: Sesame chicken salad
- Dessert: A glass of red wine and a block of very dark, bitter chocolate

Saturday

- Breakfast: Kale and blackcurrant smoothie
- Snack: Green juice

- Lunch: Sirtfood bites (because of the large meal at dinner-time)
- Snack: Green juice
- Dinner" Lamb, date, and butternut tagine
- Dessert: A glass of red wine and a block of very dark, bitter chocolate

Sunday
- Breakfast: Apple pancakes with a blackcurrant compote
- Snack: Green juice
- Lunch: The sirtfood fruit salad
- Snack: Green juice
- Dinner Delicious prawn arrabbiata spaghetti
- Dessert: A glass of red wine and a block of very dark, bitter chocolate

Don't Forget to Exercise

One of the worst aspects of changing one's diet is that many people feel that it's enough for them to get healthy, but they're missing out on a crucial aspect of their weight-loss routine—exercise!

It's important to get out and break a sweat every day because it not only burns excess energy, it also increases the metabolism, decreases the effects of oxidative stress, and strengthens the muscles in the body. Taking the time to exercise for at least 30 minutes every day to break a sweat is absolutely necessary for your weight-loss journey. If you're not the one to hit the road and go for a ten-mile run (because not many people are), still remember that any form of physical movement can be greatly beneficial to you.

People often think that they need to sign-up for expensive gym memberships to exercise, but many don't realize that even going for a walk around the neighborhood is also a remarkably effective form of exercise. Going for a walk by yourself, or with your partner, or taking your dog for a walk is a great way for you to destress in a more outdoor environment, and it increases your heart rate because you're moving.

Exercise can come in many shapes and forms, and it's absolutely crucial for you to do so. Hence, finding the right form of exercise is important. Many people love running but hate swimming, you might be the type of person that likes going for a hike instead of sitting on a bicycle seat. As long as you're taking the time to get productive movement every day, you will aid in your weight-loss process.

Chapter 6: Simple Sirtfood Recipes

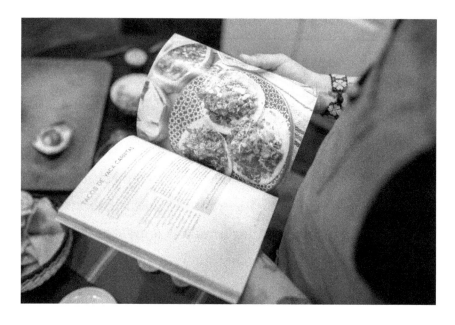

This section is going to give a myriad of different recipes to try out at home. These recipes are included because they're easy to make, high in antioxidants, low in calories, and not overly expensive. Of course, there are more expensive options for some of these recipes, and they may be nice inclusions for special occasions or just when you want to treat yourself or your family and friends.

These recipes will include preparation and cooking time, along with the servings. There will be a calorie-count in some of the recipes because most of the recipes will vary according to the specific ingredients added in.

Breakfast

#1 Scrambled Eggs and Mushrooms - The Sirtfood Style

Preparation time: 10 minutes

Cooking time: 5 minutes

Servings: 1 to 2 people

<u>Ingredients</u>

- 2 to 4 eggs
- Milk to make to the egg mixture (add as much as you desire)
- 1 to 2 teaspoons of ground turmeric
- 1 to teaspoons of mild curry powder
- 20 to 40 grams (roughly 1 to 2 ounces) of kale, roughly chopped
- 1 to 2 teaspoons of extra virgin olive oil
- 1 bird's eye chili, thinly sliced (this can be altered according to how much heat you like)
- 20 grams (roughly 1 ounce) of a white button or brown mushrooms, thinly sliced
- 5 to 10 grams (0.2 to 0.4 ounces) of parsley, finely chopped
- Any other seasonings can be added according to your own preference

Instructions

1. Mix the turmeric and curry powder in a small bowl and add a little water until you have achieved a light paste.

2. Sauté the kale for 2 to 4 minutes in a hot pan with a small drizzle of extra virgin olive oil and add salt and pepper to taste.

3. Remove the kale from the pan and heat some more oil in a frying pan over medium-to-high heat and fry the chili and mushrooms for 2 to 4 minutes until they have started to soften.

4. Remove the chili and mushroom mixture and add it to the kale.

5. Lower the heat of the pan to a low-medium heat and add your egg mixture to the pan, stirring regularly.

6. Once the eggs are cooked to your liking then add the chili, kale, and mushrooms to the scrambled eggs and serve while hot.

7. This can be enjoyed just as it is, or it can be served on a piece of rye toast, depending on the number of calories you are aiming to reach during the day.

#2 Smoked Salmon and Spinach Omelet

Preparation time: Roughly 10 minutes

Cooking time: 5 minutes

Servings: 1 to 2 people

Ingredients

- 2 to 4 large eggs (depending on how many omelets you're making)
- 100 to 200 grams (3.5 to 7 ounces) of smoked salmon, thinly sliced (tinned salmon can also be purchased if cheaper or if other variants aren't available)
- ½ to 1 teaspoon of capers
- 10 to 20 grams (0.35 to 0.7 ounces) of rocket and spinach, roughly chopped
- 1 to 2 teaspoons of fresh parsley, roughly chopped
- 1 tsp Extra virgin olive oil
- Salt and pepper to taste
- Additional chili can be added to this omelet if desired.

Instructions

1. Crack the eggs into a large bowl and whisk well and season with salt and pepper.
2. Add some water to the mixture to make it lighter (milk isn't as effective in omelets because it makes the mixture too heavy).
3. Add the salmon, capers, rocket, spinach, and parsley.
4. Heat the olive oil in a non-stick frying pan until hot.
5. Turn up the grill in your oven to high so you can hold the pan underneath the grill to cook the top of the omelet.
6. Add the egg mixture to the hot pan and, using a plastic or silicone spatula, move the mixture around the pan until it covers the pan evenly.
7. Reduce the heat and let the omelet cook through.

8. Hold the pan under the grill for a few seconds to ensure the top of the omelet cooks (be careful if your nonstick pan has plastic handles because they can melt from the direct heat).

9. Slide the spatula around the edges and roll up or fold the omelet in half to serve.

10. This can be enjoyed just as it is, or it can be served on a piece of rye toast, depending on the number of calories you are aiming to reach during the day.

#3 Muesli - The Sirtfood Style

Preparation time: Does take previous preparation because this muesli is made from scratch.

Cooking time: NA

Servings: Depends on the amount of muesli made, but this is enough for one to two servings.

Ingredients

- 20 to 40 grams (0.7 to 1.4 ounces) of buckwheat flakes
- 10 to 20 grams (0.35 to 0.7 ounces) of buckwheat puffs
- 15 to 30 grams (0.5 to 1 ounce) of coconut flakes or equal amounts of desiccated coconut
- 40 to 80 grams (1.4 to 2.8 ounces) of fresh dates, pitted and chopped into smaller pieces
- 15 to 30 (0.5 to 1 ounce) grams of walnuts, roughly chopped
- 10 to 20 grams (0.35 to 0.7 ounces) of cocoa nibs

- 100 to 250 grams (3.5 to 9 ounces) of fresh strawberries, hulled and sliced

- 100 to 200 grams (3.5 to 8 ounces) of plain Greek yogurt (or vegan alternative, such as soya or coconut yogurt)

- Extra additions can be added like raisins or walnuts according to personal tastes and preferences.

Instructions

This is one of the easiest and most time-effective breakfasts of all. All you need to do is mix all of the above ingredients together and store it away until you need it. And, only adding the yogurt and strawberries before serving.

#4 Chocolate Chip Granola Cereal

Preparation time: 30 minutes

Cooking time: 30 minutes

Servings: Eight to sixteen (depending on the size of the batch)

Calories: 244 per granola serving

Ingredients

- 200 to 400 grams (8 to 16 ounces) of raw, jumbo oats

- 50 to 100 grams (1.7 to 3.4 ounces) pecan nuts or walnuts, roughly chopped

- 3 to 6 tablespoons of extra virgin olive oil

- 20 to 40 grams (0.7 to 1.4) of unsalted butter

- 1 to 2 tablespoons of dark brown sugar or molasses

- 2 to 4 tablespoons of rice malt syrup or golden syrup (depending on availability)
- 60 to 200 grams (2 to 8 ounces) of high-quality (70%+ cocoa) dark chocolate chips

Instructions

1. Preheat the oven to 320°F (160°C) or 284°F (140°C) if your oven has a convection fan.

2. Line a large baking tray with baking parchment or a silicone sheet.

3. Mix the oats and pecan nuts/walnuts together in a large bowl.

4. In a non-stick saucepan, gently heat the extra virgin olive oil, butter, brown sugar, and syrup until the butter has melted and the sugar and syrup have completely dissolved. Ensure that there aren't any sugar granules left but do not allow it to boil.

5. Pour the syrup mixture over the oats and stir thoroughly until the oats are fully covered and sticking together.

6. Distribute the granola over the baking tray, ensuring that the mixture is even throughout, and spreading it right into the corners.

7. Bake in the oven for 20 to 30 minutes until just tinged golden brown at the edges.

8. Remove the baking tray from the oven and leave to cool on the tray completely.

9. When the granola is cool, break up any bigger lumps on the tray with your fingers and then mix in the chocolate chips, nuts and raisins if you desire.

10. Pour or scoop the granola mixture into an airtight tub or jar, and store in a cool, dark place.

11. The granola will keep for at least two weeks, depending on how well they're stored.

12. If you desire to have granola bars instead of a granola cereal that you can use as a snack at certain periods of the day, then you can cut the baked mixture before it's cooled into the rectangular sizes that you desire.

#5 The Melon and Grape Sirt-Juice

Preparation time: 10 minutes

Cooking time: 2 to 3 minutes

Servings: 1 to 2 people

Calories: 125 per glass

Ingredients

- 1 medium cucumber, peeled if preferred, but it's better to leave the skin on because of the extra chlorophyll in the skin.

- 30 to 50 grams (roughly 1 to 2 ounces) of young spinach leaves, stalks removed

- 100 to 200 grams (3.5 to 7 ounces) red seedless grapes

- 100 to 200 grams (3.5 to 7 ounces) of cantaloupe melon, peeled and deseeded

Instructions

Juices are always easy because once the prep is done, the juice is ready in a couple of minutes and ready to drink. This juice is great on mornings that you need an extra "pick me up" and it can make a great snack for another day if you want to make a large enough amount to store some in your fridge. Just don't freeze the mixture because it doesn't freeze well. Remember that although juices are tempting to use as meal replacements, they can still have a lot of hidden sugar in them. This juice for example has grapes and cantaloupe melon, both of which are very high in fructose, so it should be consumed sparingly.

#6 Matcha Green Tea Smoothie

Preparation time: 10 minutes

Cooking time: 2 to 3 minutes

Servings: 2 to 4 people

Calories: 183 per glass

Ingredients

- 2 to 3 overly ripe bananas (the riper the banana, the easier it is for it to be blended into the smoothie
- 1 to 2 cups of fat-free milk
- 2 to 4 teaspoons of matcha green tea powder
- ½ to 1 teaspoon vanilla bean paste, extract or a scrape of the seeds from a fresh vanilla pod
- 6 to 12 ice cubes

- 2 to 4 teaspoons of wild or raw honey (be careful what honey you purchase because many cheaper variants are mixed with simple syrup, and don't have all of the health benefits of raw or wild honey.

Instructions

Combine all of these ingredients into the smoothie-maker and blend until smooth. It's better not to store this smoothie and to drink it fresh. This smoothie is a better option for a meal replacement when compared to juices because it has more of the fiber from the fruits themselves and will keep one fuller for longer.

#7 Apple Pancakes with a Blackcurrant Compote

Preparation time: 20 minutes

Cooking time: 20 to 30 minutes

Servings: 4 to 6 people

Calories: 337 per serving

Ingredients for the pancakes

- 75 to 150 grams (2.5 to 5 ounces) of raw oats
- 125 to 250 grams (4.5 to 9 ounces) of plain flour
- 1 to 2 teaspoons of baking powder
- 2 to 4 tablespoons of caster sugar
- A generous pinch of salt
- 2 to 4 apples (a variant of your choice), peeled, cored, and cut into small pieces

- 1 to 2 cups of semi-skimmed milk

- 2 egg whites (Eggs should be as large as you can find, and should be refrigerated for at least an hour before mixing)

- 2 teaspoons of extra virgin olive oil

Ingredients for the compote

- 120 to 240 grams (4.2 to 8.4 ounces) of very ripe blackcurrants, washed and stalks removed

- 2 to 4 heaped tablespoons of caster sugar

- 3 to 6 tablespoons of water

Instructions

1. Before making the pancakes, it's necessary to make the compote first. Place the blackcurrants, sugar, and water in a small pan, and bring the mixture up to a simmer and cook for 10-15 minutes. The compote will reduce down and it will become thicker in consistency.

2. Place all of the dry ingredients—the flour, oats, baking powder, caster sugar, and salt in a large bowl and mix until adequately combined.

3. Mix in the pieces of apple and then whisk in the milk a little at a time until you have a smooth mixture. Don't rush this process and ensure that all of the dry parts at the bottom of the bowl get mixed into thoroughly to prevent lumps in the pancakes.

4. Beat the egg whites to stiff peaks with an electric beater (you could do it by hand with a whisk if you don't have an electric beater, and you'll develop your forearm strength in

the process) and then fold into the pancake batter. Transfer the batter to a jug to pour into a pan later on.

5. Let the mixture rest for 10 to 15 minutes.

6. Heat the extra virgin olive oil in a non-stick frying pan on medium-high heat and pour the batter into the pan.

7. Cook on both sides until golden brown and cooked in the center.

8. Remove from the heat and cook the rest of the pancakes.

9. Serve the pancakes with the blackcurrant compote drizzled over them.

This is one of those indulgences that should be reserved for special occasions. If you have these pancakes too regularly, you may struggle to lose the weight that you're aiming to.

#8 Kale and Blackcurrant Smoothie

Preparation time: 5 minutes

Cooking time: 2 to 3 minutes

Servings: 1 to 2 people

Calories: 180 per serving

Ingredients

- 2 to 3 teaspoons of raw or wild honey
- 1 to 2 cups of freshly brewed green or matcha tea
- 10 to 20 grams (0.35 to 0.7 ounces) of baby kale leaves with their stalks removed
- 1 to 2 ripe bananas

- 40 to 100 grams of blackcurrants, washed with their stalks removed
- 6 to 10 ice cubes (depending on the size of the cubes)

Instructions

1. Combine the teaspoons of honey into the green tea while it's still hot and stir until all of the honey is completely dissolved.

2. Combine all of the ingredients into a smoothie maker and blend them together.

3. Serve immediately.

Lunch

#1 Kale Salad with Turmeric Chicken and a Honey and Lime Dressing

Preparation time: 20 minutes

Cooking time: 10 minutes

Servings: 1 to 2 people

Ingredients for the chicken

- 1 to 2 tablespoon of extra-virgin olive oil or coconut oil (if you do decide to use coconut oil, just keep in mind that coconut oil is saturated fat and much higher in calories than extra virgin olive oil)
- 1 medium brown or red onion, finely diced
- 275 to 300 grams (roughly 9 ounces) of chicken mince or finely cubed chicken thighs

- 1 to 2 large garlic cloves, finely diced (this depends on how much you like garlic)
- 1 to 2 teaspoons of turmeric powder
- 2 to 3 teaspoons of lime zest
- The juice of 1 lime
- ½ teaspoon salt and 1 teaspoon of pepper

Ingredients for the salad

- 6 to 10 broccolini stalks or 2 heaped cups of broccoli florets (whichever are available and more affordable)
- 2 to 3 tablespoons pumpkin seeds
- Several large kale leaves, with their stems removed and chopped (you can decide how much kale you want to add for how big a salad you want. Kale isn't something that you can really overdo in its raw state)
- 1 medium avocado, sliced and seasoned
- 1 large handful of fresh coriander leaves, finely chopped (optional)
- 1 large handful of fresh parsley leaves, finely chopped (optional)

Ingredients for the dressing (this can be adapted according to how many greens you added into your salad—the larger the salad, the more dressing you'll need)

- 3 to 6 tablespoons lime or lemon juice (preferably freshly squeezed)
- 1 to 2 medium-sized garlic cloves, crushed, finely diced, or grated

- 3 to 6 tablespoons of extra-virgin olive oil
- 1 to 2 teaspoons of raw honey
- 1 to 2 teaspoons of wholegrain, Dijon, or English mustard (depending on how much heat you like)
- ½ teaspoon sea salt and 1 teaspoon of freshly cracked pepper to taste

Instructions

1. Heat the extra virgin olive oil in a small frying pan over medium-high heat.

2. Add the diced onion and sauté for 4 to 6 minutes, until translucent and turning slightly golden in color.

3. Add the chicken and garlic and stir for 4 to 5 minutes over medium-high heat, browning all of the meat and cooking it through, breaking it apart as it cooks.

4. Add the lime zest, lime juice, turmeric, salt, and pepper and stir through thoroughly. Allow the spices to cook with meat to release more flavor, and stir frequently for a further 4 to 5 minutes.

5. Set the cooked chicken aside.

6. While the chicken is cooling, bring a small pot of water to a boil.

7. Add the broccolini and cook for a few minutes, until the shoots are tender.

8. Rinse under cold water and cut into a few pieces each.

9. Add the pumpkin seeds to the frying pan that still has the juices from the chicken and toast over medium heat for 2 to 3 minutes. Ensure to stir frequently to prevent burning.

10. Season with a pinch of salt and pepper and set aside (If you'd prefer to use raw pumpkin seeds, they are also fine to use).

11. Place chopped kale in a salad bowl and pour the dressing over the leaves and toss and massage the kale with the dressing (this will soften the kale, kind of like what citrus juice does to fish, the acidity starts to cook the leaves).

12. Finally toss the salad with the cooked chicken, the broccolini, the fresh herbs, the pumpkin seeds, and the avocado slices.

13. Enjoy!

This meal is wholesome and can easily work for lunch or dinner. But, do remember that meals with kale and spinach leaves do take a lot of effort to digest. If you are going to eat this for supper then ensure that you still have a few hours before you go to bed.

#2 Chicken, Kale, and Buckwheat Noodles with Miso Dressing

Preparation time: 15 minutes

Cooking time: 15 minutes

Servings: 1 to 2 people

Ingredients for the chicken and noodles

- 2 to 3 large handfuls of kale leaves (cleaned, removed from the stem, and roughly cut)

- 150 - 300 grams (Roughly 5 to 10 ounces) of buckwheat noodles (ensure that you use products that are 100%

buckwheat, and try to avoid normal or refined wheat products).

- 3 to 4 shiitake mushrooms, finely sliced (shiitake mushrooms are readily available in their dried forms and can be cheaper and easier to store in this way. If you use dried shiitake mushrooms, ensure that you rehydrate them first before slicing them).

- 1 to 2 teaspoons of extra virgin olive oil or coconut oil.

- 1 medium red or brown onion, finely diced.

- 1 to 2 medium free-range chicken breasts, sliced or diced into small pieces for quick cooking.

- 1 bird's eye chili or another long red chili, thinly sliced (seeds in or out depending on how hot you want your dish. Do keep in mind that spicy foods do accelerate the metabolism, so it will be worth your while to work up to the hot stuff if you're not usually used to it).

- 2 to 3 large garlic cloves, crushed or finely diced.

- 2 to 6 tablespoons of low-sodium soy sauce.

Ingredients for the miso dressing (the amount of this dressing is entirely dependent on your taste and can be altered accordingly)

- 1½ to 3 tablespoons of fresh and organic miso paste

- 1 to 3 tablespoons of tamari sauce

- 1 to 3 tablespoons of extra-virgin olive oil

- 1 to 3 tablespoon of freshly squeezed lemon or lime juice

- 1 to 3 teaspoons of sesame oil for extra flavor (optional)

Instructions

1. Bring a medium-sized pot or saucepan of water to the boil and add a pinch of salt with the kale and cook for 1 to 2 minutes until tender and slightly wilted.

2. Remove the kale and set it aside but reserve the water that it was cooked in and bring it back to the boil. Once the water is boiling again, add the noodles and cook according to the package instructions (which is usually about 5 minutes until it's al dente).

3. Rinse under cold water and set aside.

4. While the noodles are cooling, pan fry the shiitake mushrooms in a little extra virgin olive oil or coconut oil (about a teaspoon) for 3 to four minutes, until soft and lightly browned on each side.

5. Sprinkle with sea salt, remove from the pan, and set aside.

6. In the same frying pan that you cooked the mushrooms in, heat more oil over medium-high heat.

7. Sauté the diced onion and chili for 3 to 4 minutes and then add the chicken pieces.

8. Cook the chicken pieces for 5 to 8 minutes over medium heat, stirring a couple of times. Once the chicken is thoroughly browned then add the tamari sauce, garlic, and a little splash of water.

9. Continue to cook for a further 3 to 4 minutes, ensuring that you stir frequently until chicken is cooked through.

10. Finally, add the kale and noodles and mix thoroughly with the chicken to warm up. Add the mix of miso dressing and drizzle over the noodles right at the end of cooking,

because miso is filled with probiotic cultures, and this way you will keep all those beneficial probiotics in the miso alive and active without destroying them from the heat of cooking.

11. Enjoy while it's hot!

#3 Baked Salmon Salad with Mint Dressing

Preparation time: 10 to 15 minutes

Cooking time: 15 minutes

Servings: 1 to 2 people

Calories: 340 per serving

Ingredients for the salmon salad

- 1 to 2 salmon fillets (approximately 130 grams each)
- 40 to 80 grams (1.5 to 3 ounces) of mixed salad leaves (kale, lettuce, and rocket)
- 40 to 80 grams (1.5 to 3 ounces) young spinach leaves
- 2 to 4 radishes, cleaned, trimmed, and thinly sliced
- 1 medium cucumber (around 50 grams or roughly 2 ounces), cut into chunks
- 2 to 4 spring onions, cleaned, trimmed, and sliced (depending on personal preference)
- 1 medium-sized handful of parsley, roughly chopped

Ingredients for the salad dressing

- 1 to 2 teaspoons of low-fat mayonnaise

- 2 to 4 tablespoons of natural, fat-free Greek yogurt
- 1 to 2 tablespoons of rice vinegar
- 2 to 10 mint leaves, finely chopped (depending on your affinity towards mint)
- A pinch of sea salt and one teaspoon of freshly cracked black pepper

Instructions

1. Preheat the oven to 392°F (200°C) or 356°F (180°C) if you have a convention fan in your oven.

2. Place the salmon fillets on a baking tray and season liberally with salt and pepper and bake for 15 to 20 minutes until just cooked through.

3. Remove from the oven and set aside to rest.

4. It doesn't matter if the salmon loses most of its heat because the salmon is just as nice hot or cold in this salad.

5. If your salmon has skin, don't throw it away. Simply cook the skin on the skin-side down and remove the salmon from the skin using a fish slice after cooking. Once the meat is cooked it should slide off easily enough.

6. In a medium-sized bowl, mix the rice wine vinegar, mint leaves, mayonnaise, yogurt, and salt and pepper together and leave to stand for at least ten minutes to allow the flavors to interact with each other and to develop.

7. Arrange the salad leaves of your choosing and the spinach on a serving plate and top with the sliced radishes, cucumber, spring onions, and parsley.

8. Once the salad is practically ready, flake the cooked salmon onto the salad and cover with your dressing.

9. Toss the salad and ensure that the dressing adequately coats the salad.

10. Serve and enjoy!

#4 The Fragrant Asian Hotpot

Preparation time: 10 to 15 minutes

Cooking time: 15 minutes

Servings: 1 to 2 people

Calories: 185 per serving

Ingredients

- 1 to 2 teaspoons of organic tomato purée (or just one without preservatives)
- 1 to 2 whole star anise (they can be crushed, added whole or 1/4 tsp ground anise can be added from a spice jar)
- One medium-sized handful of parsley (around 20 grams), stalks finely chopped
- A small handful of coriander (around 10 grams), stalks finely chopped
- The juice of a freshly-squeezed lime
- 500ml to 1 liter of chicken stock (it can be fresh or made with 1 cube of premade stock)
- 1 medium carrot, peeled and cut into matchsticks

- 50 to 100 grams (roughly 2 to 4 ounces) of broccoli, cut into small florets
- 50 to 100 grams (roughly 2 to 4 ounces) of bean sprouts
- 100 to 300 grams (4 to 10 ounces) of raw tiger prawns (depending on how much protein you desire)
- 100 to 300 grams (4 to 10 ounces) of firm tofu, diced into small squares
- 50 to 100 grams (2 to 4 ounces) of rice noodles or egg noodles, cooked according to packet instructions
- 50 to 100 grams (2 to 4 ounces) of cooked water chestnuts that have been drained
- 20 to 40 grams (roughly 1.5 to 3 ounces) of preserved ginger (the same kind you'd eat at a sushi bar), chopped
- 1 large tablespoon of high-quality miso paste

Instructions

1. This is a relatively easy dish to replicate, once you have all of the ingredients. First, place the tomato purée, star anise, parsley, coriander, lime juice, and chicken stock in a large saucepan or pot and bring to a simmer for at least 10 minutes (it's important to let the flavors gently interact with one another, and rushing this process can lead to a mediocre form of an Asian hotpot).

2. Add the carrot, broccoli, prawns, tofu, noodles and water chestnuts and simmer gently until the prawns are cooked through. Remove from the heat and stir in the sushi ginger and miso paste.

3. Serve sprinkled with the parsley and coriander leaves.

#5 Baked Turmeric Salmon

Preparation time: 10 to 15 minutes

Cooking time: 15 minutes

Servings: 1 to 2 people

Calories: 220 per serving

Ingredients for the salmon

- 125 to 250 grams (4.5 to 9 ounces) of skinned salmon (if you get the variant that has the skin still attached then grill it skin-side down until the skin is crispy. It's very tasty and it won't disappoint).
- 1 to 2 teaspoons of extra virgin olive oil
- 1 to 2 teaspoons of ground turmeric
- ½ cup of the juice of a lemon

Ingredients for the spicy celery

- 1 to 2 teaspoons of extra virgin olive oil
- 40 to 80 grams (roughly 1.5 to 3 ounces) of brown or red onion, finely chopped
- 60 to 120 grams (2 to 4 ounces) of tinned, green lentils
- 1 to 2 medium-sized garlic cloves, crushed or finely chopped
- 2 to 4 grams (0.1 to 0.2 ounces) of fresh ginger, finely chopped
- 1 medium-sized bird's eye chili, finely chopped
- 150 to 300 grams (5 to 10 ounces) of celery, cut into 2cm lengths

- 1 to 2 teaspoons of mild curry powder
- 130 to 250 grams (4.5 to 9 ounces) of fresh tomato, cut into wedges
- 1 cup of chicken or vegetable stock
- 1 to 2 tablespoons of fresh, chopped parsley

Instructions

1. Preheat the oven to 392°F (200°C) or 356°F (180°C) if you have a convention fan in your oven.

2. Before you bake the salmon, start with the spicy celery. Heat a frying pan over medium-low heat, and add the extra virgin olive oil until the oil is thoroughly heated.

3. Then add the onion, garlic, ginger, chili, and celery. And fry them all together gently for around 3 to 4 minutes or until soft and tender but not changing color.

4. Then add the curry powder and cook for a further minute to release all of the flavors in the curry powder.

5. Add the tomatoes and cook for a few minutes and then the stock and lentils. Simmer gently for 10 to 12 minutes. You can cook this according to your own personal preference and you may want to increase or decrease the cooking time depending on how crunchy you like your celery.

6. Place aside and start working on your salmon. Mix the turmeric, extra virgin olive oil, and lemon juice and rub over the salmon.

7. Place the salmon on a baking tray and cook for 10 to 12 minutes. Ensure that you don't overcook the fish.

8. To finish this dish, stir the parsley through the celery and serve with the salmon while the fish rests.

9. Enjoy!

#6 The Simple Chicken Salad

This recipe is great for anyone that is in a rush and wants to make a tasty recipe with some leftover chicken. This can work with any cuts of chicken, but it's best served with chicken fillets.

Preparation time: 5 minutes

Cooking time: NA because everything is already cooked

Servings: 1 to 2 people

Calories: 190 per serving

<u>Ingredients</u>

- 75 to 120 grams (2.6 to 4.2 ounces) of fat-free Greek yogurt
- The juice of 1/2 of a lemon, freshly squeezed
- 1 to 2 teaspoons of fresh coriander, finely chopped according to personal preference
- 1 to 2 teaspoons of turmeric powder
- ½ to 1 teaspoon curry powder (mild or hot according to how much heat you'd like)
- 100 to 300 grams (3.5 to 10 ounces) of previously cooked chicken breast/fillet, shredded or cut into bite-sized pieces
- 6 to 10 walnut halves, finely chopped
- 1 to 2 fresh dates, deseeded and finely chopped

- 20 to 40 grams (0.7 to 1.4 ounces) of red onion, finely diced
- 1 to 2 bird's eye chilis (personal preference)
- 40 to 80 grams (1.4 to 2.8 ounces) of rocket or baby spinach to serve

Instructions

Mix the ingredients–the yogurt, lemon juice, coriander, and spices together in a bowl. Add all the remaining ingredients and serve on a bed of the rocket. This salad can be premade and eaten as a quick lunch on-the-go. It makes a great lunch for those with busy office hours.

#7 Buckwheat with Kale and Red Onion Dhal

Preparation time: 5 minutes

Cooking time: 20 minutes

Servings: 3 to 4 people

Calories: 190 per serving

Ingredients

- 1 to 2 tablespoons of extra virgin olive oil
- 1 medium-sized red onion, finely sliced or diced
- 3 large garlic cloves, grated or crushed
- 1 inch of fresh ginger, peeled and grated
- 1 to 2 birds eye chilis, deseeded and finely chopped (this can be changed according to your own personal preference)
- 2 to 3 teaspoons of turmeric powder

- 2 to 3 teaspoons garam masala
- 160 to 200 grams (5.6 to 7 ounces) of red lentils
- 2 cups of reduced-fat coconut milk
- 1 cup of water
- 100 to 200 grams (3.5 to 7 ounces) of kale or spinach
- 160 to 200 grams (5.6 to 7 ounces) of buckwheat or brown rice

Instructions

1. Drizzle the extra virgin olive oil into a large and deep saucepan and add the diced or sliced red onion.

2. Cook on a low-medium heat for about 2 minutes, and then add the lid for 5 minutes until softened.

3. Once the onion is translucent, add the garlic, ginger, and bird's eye chili and cook for 2 more minutes to release all of the flavors (the smell of these ingredients cooking together may cause your neighbors to pop by).

4. Add the turmeric, garam masala, and a splash of water and cook for 2 more minutes (don't neglect to give the time to cook these spices, because they need the heat of the pan to release their flavors fully. Neglecting this affects the overall taste of the dhal later on).

5. Add the red lentils, 2 cups of coconut milk, and 1 cup of water. Mix everything together thoroughly and cook for around 20 to 30 minutes over low heat with the lid on (this dish needs to be cooked gently).

6. Stir occasionally and add a little more water if the dhal starts to dry-out and stick to the pan.

7. After 20 to 30 minutes add the spinach/kale. Once the leaves have wilted, stir thoroughly and replace the lid, cook for a further 5 to 6 minutes (judge accordingly, because all that needs to be cooked now is the leaves. When they're done, your dish is ready).

8. When there are around 15 minutes left before the dhal is ready, place the buckwheat or rice in a medium pot or saucepan and add salt and boiling water.

9. Bring the water back to the boil and cook for 10 to 12 minutes (or a little longer if you prefer your buckwheat less al dente).

10. Drain the buckwheat and serve with the dhal while everything is still hot.

#8 Avocado and Buckwheat Pasta Salad

Preparation time: 10 to 15 minutes (depending on whether or not you have pre-cooked buckwheat pasta available).

Cooking time: 3 to 5 minutes

Servings: 1 to 2 people

Calories: 200 per serving

Ingredients

- 50 to 100 grams (1.7 to 3.4 ounces) of uncooked buckwheat pasta. If you still need to cook the pasta, ensure that you leave the pasta to cool before adding it to the salad. Cook the pasta according to the packet instructions)

- 1 large handful of fresh rocket spinach

- 1 large handful of fresh baby spinach

- A small handful of fresh basil leaves (be sure to crush them and tear them into your salad. Don't chop them because the crushing and tearing releases the oils in the leaves and makes it much more fragrant).

- 20 to 30 grams (0.7 to 1 ounce) of ripe cherry tomatoes that have been halved

- 1 large ripe avocado, sliced or diced (lemon juice, salt, and pepper are optional for the avocado, but it's definitely recommended).

- 10 to 20 grams (0.35 to 0.70 ounces) of olives (olives are high in healthy fats, but still quite high in calories, so be sure you don't overdo the number of olives that you put into your salad).

- 1 to 2 tablespoons of extra virgin olive oil

- 20 to 30 grams (0.7 to 1 ounce) of pine nuts or roasted pumpkin seeds

Instructions

1. Gently toss and combine all of the ingredients (barring the pine nuts or pumpkin seeds) into a large bowl and sprinkle the nuts and seeds over the top.

2. Serve on a hot afternoon when you feel like something light and refreshing.

#9 Greek Salad Skewers with Mediterranean Dressing

Preparation time: 10 to 15 minutes

Cooking time: NA

Servings: 1 to 2 people

Calories: 306 per serving

Ingredients for the skewers

- 2 to 4 wooden skewers (depending on how many skewers you want to make)
- 8 to 20 large, pitted black olives
- 8 to 20 ripe cherry whole tomatoes
- 1 to 2 large, ripe yellow peppers, cut into single-inch squares
- 1 to 2 red onion, cut in half and then separated into separate pieces, or chopped into single-inch squares
- 100 to 200 grams (3.5 to 7 ounces) of cucumber, cut into single-inch pieces
- 100 to 200 grams (3.5 to 7 ounces) of feta (whichever flavor you prefer), cut into single-inch cubes

Ingredients for the dressing

- 1 to 2 tablespoons of extra virgin olive oil
- The juice of 1 lemon, freshly squeezed
- 1 to 2 teaspoons of balsamic vinegar
- 1 clove of garlic, peeled and crushed (it's better not to dice the garlic for this dressing because crushing it will enable it to infuse more generously into the dressing)

- 1 small handful of fresh basil, finely chopped
- 1 small handful of fresh oregano, finely chopped
- 1 small handful of fresh parsley, finely chopped
- ½ teaspoon of sea salt and 1 teaspoon of freshly cracked black pepper

Instructions

1. Get all of the cut salad pieces and start threading them onto the skewers, keeping them in the same order.
2. Combine all of the dressing ingredients in a bowl and cover the skewers generously.
3. Serve on a hot afternoon or at a family gathering because these skewers are always crowd-pleasers.

#10 Sesame Chicken Salad

Preparation time: 10 to 15 minutes

Cooking time: NA

Servings: 1 to 2 people

Calories: 304 per serving

Ingredients for the salad

- 1 to 2 tablespoons of sesame seeds
- 1 medium-to-large cucumber, peeled and deseeded, then sliced into half-rings
- 100 to 200 grams (3.5 to 7 ounces) of baby kale, destalked and roughly chopped

- 60 to 100 grams (2 to 3.5 ounces) of pak choi, very finely shredded (cabbage can be substituted if pak choi is unavailable)
- 1 medium-sized red onion, very finely diced or sliced
- 1 large handful of fresh parsley, roughly chopped
- 150 to 200 grams (5 to 7 ounces) of previously cooked chicken breast/fillet, finely shredded

Ingredients for the dressing

- 1 to 2 tablespoons of extra virgin olive oil
- 1 to 3 teaspoons of sesame oil (adjust according to your own flavor preference)
- The juice of 1 large lime
- 1 teaspoon of raw or wild honey (adjust according to your own flavor preference)
- 2 teaspoons of low-sodium soy sauce

Instructions

1. Before assembling the salad, toast a couple of tablespoons of sesame seeds in a dry frying pan for 2 to 3 minutes until lightly browned and very fragrant. It's important not to use oil in this process because that will ruin the toasting of the sesame seeds. Ensure the pan is completely dry before adding them. Once toasted, transfer the seeds to a plate to cool and set aside.

2. In a medium-sized bowl, mix together the extra virgin olive oil, honey, sesame oil, soy sauce, and lime juice to make the dressing.

3. Place the kale, pak choi (cabbage), cucumber, and onion in a large mixing bowl and gently toss together.

4. Pour the dressing over the salad and thoroughly mix again.

5. Distribute the salad between the plates that you are serving and top with the shredded chicken.

6. Sprinkle the sesame seeds over the salad just before serving.

Dinner

It's important to note that even though the 'Lunch' and 'Dinner' sections are separated, these recipes can be used interchangeably for each other. It's entirely up to you what meal you'd like to eat at what time of day (as long as you don't exceed the number of calories that you are aiming for).

#1 King Prawn Stirfry with Buckwheat Noodles (Asian)

Preparation time: 10 to 15 minutes

Cooking time: Around 20 minutes

Servings: 1 to 2 people

Calories: 350 per serving

Ingredients

- 150 to 300 grams (5 to 10 ounces) of deveined and shelled raw king prawns

- 2 to 5 teaspoons of tamari sauce or soy sauce (whichever you prefer and is accessible)

- 2 to 5 teaspoons of extra virgin olive oil
- 75 to 150 grams (2.5 to 5 ounces) of buckwheat noodles
- 1 to 3 large garlic cloves, crushed (preferable) or finely chopped
- 1 to 3 bird's eye chilis, finely chopped (remove the seeds if you want to make the heat less intense)
- 1 to 3 teaspoons of grated or finely chopped fresh ginger
- 20 to 40 grams (0.7 to 1.4 ounces) of red onions, thinly sliced
- 40 to 80 grams of celery, sliced into small chunks
- 75 to 100 grams (2.6 to 3.5 ounces) of green beans, chopped into 1-inch pieces
- 50 to 100 grams (1.8 to 3.5 ounces) of kale, destalked and roughly chopped
- ½ to 1 cup of chicken stock
- 10 grams (0.35 ounces) of lovage or celery leaves (whichever is easiest to come by)

Instructions

1. Heat a drizzle of extra virgin olive in a non-stick frying pan over medium-high heat, and then cook the prawns.
2. Once the prawns have been in the pan for a couple of minutes, add in the tamari/soy sauce and an extra drizzle of extra virgin olive oil. Continue cooking for 3 to 4 minutes.
3. Transfer the prawns to a plate and set aside for later.

4. Wipe the pan out because you're going to use it again for the rest of the stir-fry.

5. Bring a pot or saucepan of water to the boil and cook the buckwheat noodles in salted, boiling water for as long as directed on the packet.

6. Once the noodles are cooked, drain them and set them aside.

7. While the noodles are boiling, fry the ginger, garlic, chili, kale, red onion, celery, and beans in the remaining oil in your non-stick pan over medium-high heat until all of the vegetables are tender.

8. Once they're tender add the stock and bring the mixture to the boil and then turn down the heat.

9. Simmer the mixture for an additional minute or two, so that the vegetables don't overcook and are still crunchy.

10. Once you're satisfied that everything is cooked, add the prawns and buckwheat noodles and mix thoroughly.

11. Finally, add lovage/celery leaves to the pan, and bring the mixture back to the boil to quickly wilt the leaves.

12. Remove from the heat and serve immediately.

#2 A Fragrant Asian Hotpot

Preparation time: 10 to 15 minutes

Cooking time: Around 10 minutes

Servings: 2 people

Calories: 185 per serving

Ingredients

- 2 teaspoons of tomato purée or 1 teaspoon of tomato paste because it's more concentrated

- 2 star anise, finely crushed or ground (or 1/4 tsp ground anise)

- One medium-sized handful of fresh parsley, with the stalks and leaves, finely chopped

- One small handful of fresh coriander, with the stalks and leaves, finely chopped

- The juice of 1 medium-sized lime

- 2 cups of chicken stock (can be fresh or made with 1 cube and 2 cups of boiling water)

- 1 large carrot, peeled and cut into small matchstick sizes

- 30 to 50 grams (roughly 1 to 2 ounces) of broccoli, cut into small, bite-sized florets

- 30 to 50 grams (roughly 1 to 3 ounces) of bean sprouts

- 100 to 200 grams (4 to 8 ounces) of raw tiger prawns, that are shelled and deveined (this can be substituted with king prawns if you prefer)

- 100 to 200 grams (4 to 8 ounces) of firm tofu, chopped into small cubes

- 50 to 100 grams (2.3 to 4.6 ounces) of rice noodles (cook the noodles according to the instructions on the packet)

- 30 to 50 grams (roughly 1 to 3 ounces) of cooked water chestnuts (ensure that they're completely drained before adding them to the mixture)

- 10 to 20 grams (0.35 to 0.7 ounces) of pickled ginger, chopped into small pieces
- 2 tablespoons of high-quality miso paste

Instructions

1. Add the tomato paste or purée, coriander, parsley, star anise, lime juice and chicken stock in a large saucepan and bring to a boil.

2. Once boiling, reduce the heat and simmer for 10 to 15 minutes.

3. Add the prawns, broccoli, carrot, noodles, tofu, and water chestnuts to the mixture and simmer gently until the prawns completely are cooked through.

4. Once cooked, remove the saucepan from the heat and stir in the miso paste and pickled ginger.

5. Serve immediately and sprinkle with extra parsley and coriander leaves if you so desire.

#3 Lamb, Date, and Butternut Tagine

Preparation time: 20 minutes

Cooking time: 1 hour and 30 minutes

Servings: 4 people

Calories: 330 per serving

Ingredients

- 2 to 3 tablespoons of extra virgin olive oil
- 1 large red onion, sliced into chunks (can be thin slices if you prefer)
- 1 inch of fresh ginger, peeled and grated
- 3 to 5 large garlic cloves, sliced, grated, or crushed
- 1 to 3 teaspoons of bird's eye chili flakes (adjust for what type of heat intensity that you're partial towards)
- 3 teaspoons of cumin seeds, or 2 teaspoons of cumin powder
- 1 teaspoon of cinnamon powder or 1 large cinnamon stick
- 2 to 3 teaspoons of ground turmeric
- 1 kilogram (2.2 pounds) of lamb neck fillet, cut into 1-inch chunks
- 1 teaspoon of sea salt and 2 teaspoons of freshly cracked black pepper
- 100 to 200 grams (3.5 to 7 ounces) of fresh dates, pitted and chopped (the more dates you add, the sweeter and richer the sauce will become)
- 500 gram (17-ounce) can of chopped or whole tomatoes, plus an additional half a can of water
- 500 to 700 grams (17 to 25 ounces) butternut squash, chopped into 1-inch cubes
- 500 gram (17-ounce) tin of chickpeas, completely drained and rinsed through to get rid of the polysaccharides around the peas.

- 2 to 3 heaped tablespoons of fresh coriander (plus extra for garnish)
- Buckwheat, couscous, flatbreads, or rice to serve (the choice is entirely up to you)

Instructions

1. Before preparing the meal itself, it's important to preheat your oven to 284ºF (140º C).

2. Drizzle about 3 tablespoons of extra virgin olive oil into a tagine pot, large ovenproof saucepan, or cast-iron casserole dish.

3. Add the sliced onion to the dish and cook on medium-low heat with the lid on, for about 5 to 6 minutes. You want the onions to sweat and you'll see that when the onions are softened but not brown.

4. Add the turmeric, cinnamon, cumin, chili, garlic, and ginger to the sweating onions and allow the flavors to enhance. Stir well and cook for about 3 more minutes with the lid off. Remember that the spices need time to enhance and they need the heat to do so. Avoid adding water unnecessarily, but do add a splash of water if it gets too dry. You don't want it to burn

5. Once the spices have been cooked thoroughly, then it's time to add in the lamb chunks. Stir the mixture well to coat the meat in the onions and spices and then add the salt when the lamb chunks have started browning. Then add the chopped dates and the can of tomatoes including at least half a can of water (which equates to 1 cup).

6. Bring the lamb tagine to the boil and then lower the heat and allow it to simmer for 5 minutes. Then put the lid on the dish and place it in your preheated oven for 1 hour and 30 minutes (this time can be adjusted if you want to cook it longer for more tender meat, but then the heat must just be slightly reduced to prevent the lamb tagine from drying out).

7. When the lamb has been cooking for around an hour and there are thirty minutes left before the end of the cooking time, add in the butternut pieces and washed chickpeas.

8. Stir everything together, and ensure that all of the butternut pieces are covered with liquid, and then put the lid back on and return the dish back into the oven for the final 30 minutes of cooking.

9. When the lamb tagine is ready, remove it from the oven and stir through the chopped coriander.

10. This dish can be served with practically any starch, but it's best to choose one like buckwheat because it promotes the highest sirtuin production. But you can serve it with buckwheat, couscous, flatbreads or basmati rice.

You may have read this recipe and thought that you loved the sound of it, but you don't own a cast-iron dish or oven-proof saucepan. If this is the case, then simply cook the lamb tagine in a regular saucepan until it has to go in the oven. When it's ready then you can transfer the ingredients into a regular casserole dish before placing in the oven (just ensure it's one with a lid). Once the casserole dish goes into the oven, you should add an extra 5 to 10 minutes of cooking time to allow for the fact that the casserole dish will need extra time to heat up because it went into the oven relatively cold.

#4 Delicious Prawn Arrabbiata Spaghetti

Preparation time: 40 minutes

Cooking time: 30 minutes

Servings: 1 to 2 people

Calories: 350 per serving

Ingredients for the pasta

- 150 to 200 grams (5 to 7 ounces) of raw shelled, deveined prawns (ideally king prawns but other prawns will do)
- 60 to 100 grams (2 to 3.5 ounces) of buckwheat pasta
- 2 to 3 tablespoons of extra virgin olive oil

Ingredients for the arrabbiata sauce

- 1 medium-sized red onion, finely chopped
- 2 to 3 large garlic cloves, crushed, grated, or finely chopped
- 30 to 50 grams (1 to 1.7 ounces) of fresh celery, finely diced or chopped
- 1 to 3 bird's eye chilis, finely chopped (adjust according to how much heat you like)
- 1 to 2 teaspoons of dried mixed herbs
- 2 teaspoons of extra virgin olive oil
- ½ cup of crisp white wine (optional, but it does promote the flavor of the sauce as it cooks away)
- 500 gram (17-ounce) tin of chopped tomatoes
- 1 small handful of fresh chopped parsley

Instructions

1. Heat a drizzle of extra virgin olive oil in a non-stick pan over medium-high heat and fry the onion and dried herbs together for about 2 minutes. Once the onions have started to become more translucent then add the garlic, celery, and chili. Cook all of the ingredients in the olive oil for an extra 2 to 3 minutes.

2. Once the ingredients are well sautéed, turn the heat up a little higher to medium, and add the wine and cook for 2 to 3 minutes.

3. Add the can of tomatoes and leave the sauce to simmer without the lid on over medium-low heat for 15 to 30 minutes. Judge this according to how the sauce is responding to the heat, but you want to aim until it has a nice rich consistency. If you feel the sauce is getting too thick simply add a little water.

4. While the sauce is simmering and all of the flavors are interacting with one another, bring a large pot of salted water to the boil and cook the pasta according to the packet instructions.

5. When the pasta is cooked to your liking (hopefully al dente), drain the pasta and toss it with the olive oil, extra dried herbs, and freshly cracked black pepper and keep in the pan until needed.

6. Ensure that the prawns have turned opaque in the middle before turning off the heat. Once they're cooked add the fresh parsley and serve (if you are using cooked prawns add them with the parsley, bring the sauce to a gentle simmer for 3 to 4 minutes and serve).

7. Add the cooked pasta to the sauce, mix thoroughly but without breaking the noodles, and serve.

#5 Chargrilled Steak with a Red Wine Jus, Herb Roasted Potatoes, Onion Rings, and Garlic Kale

Preparation time: 30 minutes

Cooking time: 30 minutes

Servings: 1 to 2 people

Calories: 365 per serving

Ingredients

- 200 to 300 grams (7 to 10 ounces) of baby potatoes, peeled and cut into 1-inch cubes (it's better to cook with baby potatoes because they have a lower GI than large potatoes)
- 1 to 2 tablespoons of extra virgin olive oil
- One medium-sized handful of parsley (10 grams), finely chopped
- 1 medium-sized red onion, diced very finely
- 100 grams (3.5 ounces) of kale, destalked and finely chopped
- 2 to 3 garlic cloves, crushed, grated, or finely chopped
- Steaks of your choice (it's advisable to look for sirloin or rump because of their lower fat content, but do ensure that they're at least an inch thick)
- ¼ cup of dry red wine
- ½ cup of beef stock
- 2 teaspoons of tomato purée or 1 teaspoon of tomato paste

- 2 teaspoons of corn flour, dissolved in 2 tablespoons of water

Instructions

1. Before you get started on your meal preparation, heat the oven to 356°F (180°C).

2. Place the baby potatoes in a large pot of salted boiling water, and cook for 8 to 10 minutes, and then drain (the potatoes will still be undercooked but the rest of the cooking process will occur in the oven).

3. Place the potatoes in a roasting tray with 3 teaspoons of extra virgin olive oil, season generously with sea salt, black pepper, and mixed herbs, and roast in the hot oven for 30 to 40 minutes. It's important to turn the potatoes every 10 minutes to ensure even browning on the skin and cooking on all sides.

4. When cooked, remove the baby potatoes from the oven, and sprinkle with the chopped parsley and mix well.

5. Set aside for later.

6. Heat an extra drizzle of extra virgin olive oil in a non-stick saucepan and sauté the chopped onion in the olive oil over medium heat for 5 to 8 minutes, until soft and nicely caramelized. Once the onions have started to brown, turn the heat down and keep them warm on very low heat.

7. Steam the kale in the microwave or in a pot with little water for 3 to 4 minutes and then drain off any excess liquid.

8. Sauté the garlic on low heat in ½ teaspoon of extra virgin olive oil for about 1 minute, so that it's soft but not browned. Add the steamed kale and fry for a further couple

of minutes, until completely tender. Reduce the heat and keep warm for later.

9. Heat a cast-iron steak pan on high heat on the stove until it's smoking. While the pan is heating up, take the time to prepare your steaks. There are numerous dry-rubs that are available in the grocery store, but since this meal is relatively simple, the best way to flavor these steaks is with three ingredients only—extra virgin olive oil, coarse sea salt, and freshly cracked black pepper.

10. Leave the steaks in the oil mixture for a few minutes as the pan heats up, and when it's searingly hot, pop the steak/s down on the surface of the pan. If it isn't sizzling when it touches the metal then it's not hot enough! Let the steaks cook for 1 minute on each side, and don't move them unless you're turning them. Cook the steaks between 5 and 8 minutes for a delicious medium-rare cook (you can adjust the time if you need to, but medium-rare is, by far, the superior way to eat it.

11. Once the steaks are cooked, remove the meat from the pan and set aside to rest (resting is important because it keeps the delicious juices of the meat within it. As the pan is cooling, add the wine to the still-hot pan to bring up any meat residue. Cook until the wine is reduced by half, until syrupy and with a concentrated wine flavor.

12. After the wine has become a delicious syrup, add the stock and tomato purée to the steak pan and bring to the boil. Once boiling, lower the heat to a gentle simmer and then add the corn flour paste to thicken your sauce, adding it a little at a time until you have your desired consistency. As your steaks rest, they'll release some juices onto the plate that they're resting on... don't let those juices go to waste!

Stir in any of the juices from the rested steak into the thickened wine jus and serve with the rest of the meal items.

13. This is definitely a meal worth keeping for a special occasion or when you're trying to impress your date.

Snacks

#1 The Sirtfood Snack

This recipe is designed to give you a little "pick me up" when you're feeling very depleted of energy, and although celery sticks and carrots work well, this snack is designed to help in times of desperate need and exhaustion.

Ingredients

- 150 to 200 grams (roughly 5 to 7 ounces) of walnuts or pecan nuts
- 30 to 50 grams (roughly 1 to 2 ounces) of very dark chocolate (at least 80% cocoa solids), broken into pieces.
- 10 grams (0.35 ounces) of cocoa nibs (these can be increased if you want to forgo the chocolate component completely.
- 200 to 400 grams (7 to 14 ounces)of fresh dates, pitted and cut into small pieces
- 1 heaped tablespoon of high-quality cocoa powder
- 1 heaped tablespoon of ground turmeric (it may sound strange but this addition works excellently with the cocoa.

- 2 tablespoons of extra virgin olive oil (add more if the mixture is still too dry and can't be rolled into a ball)
- Vanilla seeds or 1 teaspoon of vanilla extract
- 2 tablespoons of water

Instructions

1. Place the walnuts/pecan nuts and chocolate and cocoa nibs in a food processor and process until you have a fine powder. This is one of the reasons why having very dark chocolate is necessary because it doesn't have the fat from the cocoa butter and can be ground relatively easily.

2. Once you've made your dry mixture, add all the other ingredients (barring the water) and blend until the mixture forms a ball. The water is only there as a backup and you may or may not have to add the water depending on the consistency of the mixture.

3. Roll the mixture in your hands to form balls the size of golf balls.

4. If you'd like a variation to the balls, you could roll some of them in cocoa or desiccated coconut.

5. Don't make more than you will eat in a week because they will only keep for that amount of time in your fridge.

Conclusion

There may be several doubts surrounding the sirtfood diet because of its extreme calorie restrictions, but when employed carefully and with the right number of calories, it can definitely be a worthy lifestyle choice. This book is merely the beginning of a journey that you're going to take, and even though it may be a challenging one, it's going to be one that you'll forever be grateful for. This diet was originally started to be a 21-day journey, but when used correctly, it can be used for much longer than that.

Sirtfoods will help produce the sirtuins within your cells and your cells will become more healthy because of it. You will start looking after your body from the inside out, and you'll start the process at a cellular level.

This process will be difficult in the beginning, and your mind will fight you in the beginning stages. Unfortunately, a person's mind can be their greatest enemy, because psychologically, people don't like change. Going on a diet like this is going to feel like a huge adjustment, and your mind is going to fight it in the beginning, but it will become easier when it starts to become more of a routine. If you know that you're going to struggle then it will be worthwhile to have someone that can either hold you accountable or go on this journey with you.

It's important to enjoy this process and note to see it as a diet. The moment someone starts to think that they're dieting, they will inevitably want it to end, which will leave all of their hard work undone. The sirtfood diet can become a very healthy lifestyle and can still offer tasty food and meal options. The problem with most diets is that they're boring, and can be quite bland. If, however, you are still able to enjoy the food that you eat, while helping your metabolism and effectively losing weight and then maintaining a healthy BMI, then it's definitely a worthwhile lifestyle change.

During this process, it's important to exercise regularly to help boost your metabolism and burn excess stores of glycogen and body fat. It's true that exercise and healthy eating can help boost the metabolism individually, but when combined, they will work much more effectively at reaching your goal weight and health status.

It's important for you to enjoy life and enjoy the food that you eat. If you're not going to enjoy a journey then you won't carry on with it. Cook delicious meals with the recipes provided, practically all of them have all of the ingredients that you can find at your local grocery store.

Lose the weight that you want to, and become the healthy version of yourself that you've always wanted. It's never too late to start something new, so why not go for something that will benefit you as a person.

References

Bauer, S. (2020, October 30). *What You Need to Know about the Sirtfood Diet.* https://www.shape.com/weight-loss/food-weight-loss/why-everyone-talking-about-sirtfood-diet

Baum, I. (2020, October 28). *Inside the Sirtfood Celebrity Diet Trend That's Taking Over the US.* Men's Health. https://www.menshealth.com/weight-loss/a19540610/sirtfood-diet-what-you-need-to-know/

Davis, M. (2017, June 3). *10 Health Benefits of Drinking Red Wine That Will Keep You Healthy.* Whitehall Lane. https://whitehalllane.com/10-health-benefits-of-drinking-red-wine-that-will-keep-you-healthy/

Elysium Health. (n.d.). *The Science of Sirtuins.* Our Core Science. https://www.elysiumhealth.com/en-us/science-101/why-sirtuins-are-important-for-aging

Jones, T. (2020, September 30). *The Sirtfood Diet: A Detailed Beginners Guide.* Evidence-Based. Nutrition. https://www.healthline.com/nutrition/sirtfood-diet

Krstic, Z. (2020, October 26). *What Is the Sirtfood Diet? Inside Adele's Reported Weight Loss Program.* https://www.goodhousekeeping.com/health/diet-nutrition/a30447497/what-is-sirtfood-diet/

Link, R. (2020, February 25). *7 Proven Ways Matcha Tea Improves Your Health.* Evidence Based Nutrition. https://www.healthline.com/nutrition/7-benefits-of-matcha-tea

O'Conner, A. (2006, November 28). *The Claim: Spicy Foods Increase Metabolism.* The New York Times.

https://www.nytimes.com/2006/11/28/health/nutrition/28real.html#:~:text=Generally%2C%20studies%20have%20shown%20that,also%20increase%20feelings%20of%20satiety.

Pallauf, K. (2013, August 28). *Nutrition and Healthy Ageing: Calorie Restriction or Polyphenol-Rich "MediterrAsian" Diet.* US National Library of Medicine. https://www.ncbi.nlm.nih.gov/pmc/articles/PMC3771427/

Proudfoot, J. (2020, August 28). *Adele Credits the Sirtfood Diet with Her Weight Loss, But What Does It Actually Entail?* Marie Claire. https://www.marieclaire.co.uk/life/health-fitness/the-sirtfood-diet-22576

Sirtfood Diet. (n.d.). *The Best Sirtfood Recipes.* https://sirtfooddiet.net/best-sirtfood-recipes/

Sleep Health Foundation. (n.d.). *Insomnia.* https://www.sleephealthfoundation.org.au/pdfs/Insomnia.pdf

Smith, C. (2018, November 8). *10 Health Benefits of Onions.* Facty Health. https://facty.com/food/nutrition/10-health-benefits-of-onions/?style=quick&utm_source=adwords&adid=340239079859&ad_group_id=59044642015&utm_medium=c-search&utm_term=&utm_campaign=FH-ZA---Search---aynamic-ads-(South-Africa)---desktop&gclid=Cj0KCQiA7qP9BRCLARIsABDaZzj-vmvSTyh3nMTOs3ZqLfcKP-22GQo2O-bWf6V_AaK65Hpb5WEoIvsaAmy6EALw_wcB

Warrior Coffee. (2020, 5 October). *12 Health Benefits and 6 Disadvantages of Coffee - Smashing It!*

https://blog.warriorcoffee.com/blog/12-health-benefits-and-6-disadvantages-of-coffee-smashing-it

Yan, L. (2013). *Dark Green Leafy Vegetables*. Agricultural Research Service. https://www.ars.usda.gov/plains-area/gfnd/gfhnrc/docs/news-2013/dark-green-leafy-vegetablcs/#:~:text=The%20vitamin%20K%20contents%20of,the%20best%20cancer%2Dpreventing%20foods.

CPSIA information can be obtained
at www.ICGtesting.com
Printed in the USA
LVHW080812171220
674086LV00047B/67